Benjamin Silliman
and his Circle

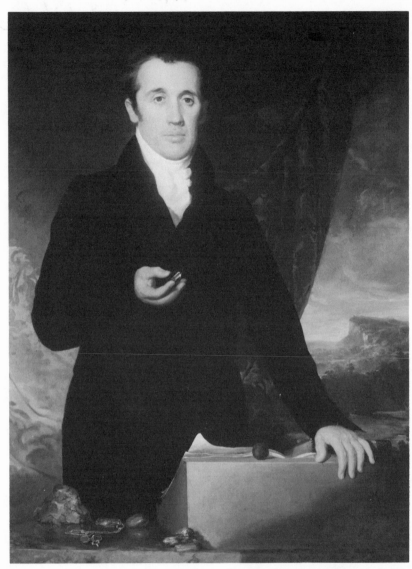

Benjamin Silliman, by Samuel F. B. Morse.

Benjamin Silliman and his Circle:

Studies on The Influence of Benjamin Silliman on Science in America

PREPARED IN HONOR OF

ELIZABETH H. THOMSON

edited by

Leonard G. Wilson

SCIENCE HISTORY PUBLICATIONS

NEW YORK

1979

Published by
Science History Publications
a division of
Neale Watson Academic Publications, Inc.
156 Fifth Avenue, New York 10010

Printed in U.S.A.

Library of Congress Cataloging in Publication Data
Main entry under title:

Benjamin Silliman and his circle.

   Bibliography: p.
   Includes index.
   CONTENTS: Wilson, L. G. Benjamin Silliman—
Greene, J. C. Protestantism, science, and
American enterprise.—Beckham, S. D. Colonel
George Gibbs. [etc.]
   1. Silliman, Benjamin, 1779-1864—Addresses,
essays, lectures.   2. Scientists—United States—
Biography—Addresses, essays, lectures.   3. Science
—United States—History—Addresses, essays,
lectures. I. Thomson, Elizabeth Harriet, 1907-
II. Wilson; Leonard Gilchrist, 1928-
Q143.S54B46   509'.22 [B]   77-21564
ISBN 0-88202-174-5

Contents

Illustrations

Preface

THIS BOOK has been prepared in honor of Elizabeth H. Thomson who retired in 1972 from the Department of History of Science and Medicine, Yale University School of Medicine. Instead of the usual festschrift, our aim was to prepare a group of related essays that would contribute to historical understanding of Benjamin Silliman in whom Elizabeth Thomson has been so long and so deeply interested.

At Yale Miss Thomson held the formal title of Research Associate, but such a title hardly describes the range of her scholarly work in the history of medicine and science, nor the multitude of ways in which she encouraged both medical students and graduate students in historical research. Author, editor of the *Journal of the History of Medicine and Allied Sciences*, friend and adviser to both faculty and students, Miss Thomson has always been especially helpful to those engaged in historical research on Benjamin Silliman.

In 1947, not long after Miss Thomson was appointed at Yale by the late Dr. John F. Fulton, then Sterling Professor of Physiology, Dr. Fulton and Miss Thomson published their excellent short biography of Benjamin Silliman—still the only modern general study of Silliman. In her research for the Silliman biography Miss Thomson developed a deep knowledge of the Silliman family papers, the papers of James Dwight Dana, and the papers of others among Silliman's colleagues and students, in the rich manuscript collections of Yale. From such knowledge she has been able to provide useful suggestions to any historian interested in Silliman, in Silliman's immediate associates, or in that far-flung group whom Silliman influenced in one way or another through his teaching at Yale, his public lectures, or the *American Journal of Science*.

The present book arose from a suggestion by Whitfield J. Bell, Jr., Executive Officer and Librarian of the American Philosophical Society at Philadelphia. The plan for it was worked out by the editor and Mr. Bell together. The editor then wrote to the various scholars, whose historical research was connected in some way with Benjamin Silliman, to explain the plan of the book and to ask them to contribute. The response was prompt and exceedingly generous. Each of the contributors has not only written an essay especially for the book, but each essay, with the exception of the editor's brief biographical sketch of Silliman, embodies fresh historical research.

Our intent has been to study Silliman's influence on the development of science in the United States through his students and junior colleagues at Yale in the early years, through the *American Journal of Science*, and through the development of the Sheffield Scientific School

ix

and graduate education in science at Yale near the close of Silliman's life. We wished to emphasize Silliman's broad national influence on science and education, but to do so by a series of essays, mainly biographical, on Silliman and some of the men and institutions he influenced most directly.

The contributors have acknowledged the various libraries and archives that have permitted the use of their manuscript collections. The editor, in compiling the list of manuscript sources for the whole book, is especially indebted to the following: Judith A. Schiff, Chief Research Archivist, Manuscripts and Archives, Yale University Library; Martin Schmitt, Special Collections, University of Oregon Library; Murphy D. Smith, Associate Librarian, American Philosophical Society Library; Katherine Thompson, Reference Assistant, State Historical Society of Wisconsin; and the Newport Historical Society. At Yale some manuscript collections have been transferred from former locations to the university library and rearranged. Judith A. Schiff, Chief Research Archivist, took the entire list of Yale manuscripts and checked it completely with the present arrangement of the collections. In addition to the research and writing of her two essays, Gloria Robinson located and obtained permission to reproduce portraits of James Dwight Dana, George Gibbs, Edward Hitchcock, Charles Upham Shepard, and Benjamin Silliman. Dr. Robinson has also helped with any question that required reference to the Yale University Library or its manuscript collections. Louis Kuslan located previously unpublished portraits of Benjamin Silliman, Jr. as a young man and his wife, Susan Forbes Silliman; and the owner, Edwin Pugsley, generously gave permission to reproduce them. I am grateful to my secretary Mrs. Helen Mammen who has typed portions of the manuscript, retyped others, and has helped in multitudinous ways.

Finally I am indebted most deeply to my wife, Adelia K. Wilson, who, in addition to constant support and encouragement, has copy edited the whole book and has prepared the bibliography and index. Without her help the book might not have appeared at all; it certainly would have been in a more ragged form.

Leonard G. Wilson
Minneapolis, Minnesota
June 1977

Benjamin Silliman:
A Biographical Sketch

LEONARD G. WILSON

BENJAMIN SILLIMAN was not a great scientific discoverer, but he was a great teacher. Both at Yale and throughout the United States, he was important primarily for the influence that he exerted upon his friends and students. Silliman taught not only those who attended his classes in Yale College, but also the readers and contributors of the *American Journal of Science*, the audiences to whom he lectured in many American cities for more than twenty years, and the readers of his textbook of chemistry and two travel works. Silliman established the teaching of the natural sciences as an integral part of the education given to students in Yale College in the early nineteenth century, and the example set by Yale was followed later by other American colleges and universities.

When Pres. Timothy Dwight appointed Benjamin Silliman professor of chemistry and natural history at Yale College in 1802, the college curriculum in America, as at Oxford and Cambridge in England, was confined entirely to the study of the Greek and Latin classics and to theology. When Silliman retired from teaching at Yale in 1853, not only were such subjects as chemistry, geology, mineralogy, and natural history part of the studies of Yale undergraduates, as they had been for half a century, but Yale also possessed a Department of Philosophy and the Arts, with professors of agricultural chemistry, practical chemistry, and civil engineering. The Department of Philosophy and the Arts was, among other things, giving students practical laboratory training in chemistry to enable them to become professional scientists. By the time of Silliman's death in 1864, slightly more than ten years later, the Yale Department of Philosophy and the Arts had become the Sheffield Scientific School and Yale had awarded the first Ph.D. degrees given in America. The Sheffield Scientific School was staffed largely with Silliman's former students and Silliman had exerted his influence to help the new school overcome successive obstacles at each stage of its development. Through the Sheffield Scientific School, Benjamin Silliman was a principal founder of graduate education in science in America. Graduate education in science at American universities in turn has created the cadre of professional research scientists who have been responsible for American scientific achievements of the succeeding century.

1

Silliman's influence extended beyond Yale to other universities. Andrew Dickson White, first president of Cornell University, was educated at Yale, and White made science teaching and scientific research an integral part of the Cornell program. Similarly Daniel Coit Gilman, first president of both the University of California and Johns Hopkins University, was a student at Yale and from 1855 to 1872 a member of the faculty, first of the Yale Scientific School and after 1861 of the Sheffield Scientific School. At Johns Hopkins, Gilman made scientific training and scientific research prominent features of the new graduate university, with rapid and important consequences for the development of scientific research in the United States. In 1869 White and Gilman helped Charles William Eliot in the preparation of his inaugural address as president of Harvard College, that address in which Eliot set forth the blueprint that was to make Harvard a university—a university in which graduate education would be offered in many departments and in which scientific training and research would become especially important.

Benjamin Silliman was born during the American Revolution on 8 August 1779 at North Stratford (now Trumbull), Connecticut, the second son of Gold Selleck Silliman and Mary Fish Silliman. At the time of Benjamin's birth, his father, a general in the Continental Army, was a prisoner of the British on Long Island, having been captured in his house at Holland Hill, Connecticut the night of the preceding first of May. A year later, in May 1780, General Silliman was released by the British authorities, and returned home to Holland Hill. There in a comfortable New England farmhouse, overlooking Long Island Sound, Benjamin Silliman spent his boyhood. In 1790 when Benjamin was only eleven, his father died leaving his mother with two boys to educate and a considerable farm to manage. Mrs. Silliman sent Benjamin and his brother Selleck to be tutored by their neighbor, the Reverend Andrew Eliot, to prepare them to enter Yale College at New Haven. In September 1792, at the age of thirteen, Benjamin Silliman entered Yale College, where in September 1796, at the age of seventeen, he was graduated A.B. He returned home to spend the year 1796–97 caring for the farm at Holland Hill.

The following year, 1797–98, Silliman taught in a private school at Wethersfield, Connecticut, but sometime during the year he decided to become a lawyer like his father and grandfather before him. In October 1798 he and his brother Selleck returned to New Haven where they entered the law office of the Honorable Simeon Baldwin as apprentices. In 1799 while Silliman was still a law student, Pres.

Timothy Dwight of Yale, an old friend of Silliman's father, appointed Benjamin a tutor in Yale College. During the next three years Silliman combined the duties of a Yale tutor with the study of law. In July 1801 Dr. Dwight invited Benjamin Silliman to become the first professor of chemistry and natural history at Yale, and after some hesitation, because he knew little of either subject, Silliman accepted. On 7 September 1802, after Silliman had passed his legal examinations, the Yale Corporation appointed him professor of chemistry and natural history in Yale College.

Silliman's first task as a young professor, twenty-three years of age, was to learn something of the principal subject, chemistry, that he had undertaken to teach. In November 1802 he went to Philadelphia where Prof. James Woodhouse taught chemistry in the medical school at the University of Pennsylvania. There, Silliman attended Professor Woodhouse's lectures. At Mrs. Smith's boarding house at the corner of Dock and Walnut streets, he met several other young men, one of whom, Robert Hare, was also studying chemistry. Hare and Silliman performed chemical experiments with the oxyhydrogen blowpipe which Hare had developed just the year before. Silliman occasionally attended lectures at the medical school by such other professors as Benjamin Rush on medicine, Benjamin Smith Barton on botany, and Caspar Wistar on anatomy and surgery. Silliman found Wistar's lectures particularly interesting, and Wistar invited Silliman to dine at his house where the Reverend Joseph Priestley, the discoverer of oxygen, was also a guest.

On his return to New Haven in March 1803 Silliman resumed his duties as a tutor in Yale College. The following November he returned to Philadelphia to study chemistry and anatomy until March 1804. In April 1804 the twenty-five-year-old professor began his first course of lectures on chemistry at Yale. He set up a chemical laboratory and the following October began to teach chemistry to his first class of seniors.

In September 1804 the Yale Corporation voted to spend $10,000 in Europe for books for the library, and chemical and other scientific apparatus. When Silliman heard of the proposed expenditure, he suggested to the Yale authorities that they send him to England to do the purchasing. Silliman pointed out that if Yale would give him the five percent commission that they would otherwise pay an agent, the sum would probably pay his travel expenses, and he might be able to learn a great deal about the sciences he was to teach. The president and fellows of Yale accepted the proposal and on 6 April 1805 Silliman sailed from New York for Liverpool to spend a year in Britain.

When Silliman landed on 3 May 1805 he found England under the threat of invasion by Napoleon's armies. After landing at Liverpool, he went to Manchester where he visited Manchester College and called on the Quaker chemist John Dalton, then in the course of developing his atomic theory. From Manchester, Silliman traveled by way of the Peak district to London where he delivered his various letters of introduction and spent much time sightseeing. Among many activities, he admired St. Paul's Cathedral, visited the Tower of London and Westminster Abbey, dined at Benjamin West's house, and visited an exhibition of paintings at Somerset House. Later, he heard the prime minister, William Pitt, speak at the House of Commons. As a visiting scientist Silliman naturally attended a *conversazione* at the house of Sir Joseph Banks, president of the Royal Society, where he met James Watt, William Hyde Wollaston, Henry Cavendish, and other noteworthy British scientists. In pursuit of his main purpose, Silliman visited instrument makers to order scientific apparatus for Yale, and booksellers to buy books for the Yale library. One day, from a shop window in the Strand, he saw Lord Nelson walking in the street, accompanied by his chaplain and followed by a crowd.

On 26 August Silliman set out on a tour of the Southwest of England to visit the tin and copper mines of Cornwall. He traveled mainly by stagecoach and visited Windsor, Bath, Bristol, Taunton, and Exeter en route. On his return journey along the south coast, Silliman visited Stonehenge and, from Southampton, crossed to the Isle of Wight. After making a circuit of the island, mostly along the beach on horseback, he crossed on 14 September from Cowes to Portsmouth in a passage boat. The boat sailed close to the British fleet of some sixty or seventy ships lying at anchor at Spithead. Off St. Helens, Silliman saw Nelson's flagship, the *Victory*, at its mooring. After they landed at Portsmouth Silliman watched Nelson embark from the beach in his barge. The crowd cheered and Nelson replied by waving his hat. After a brief visit to Holland at the end of September, Silliman returned to London and on 6 November was listening to a case in the Court of Admiralty at Doctor's Commons when the news came of Nelson's great victory at Trafalgar on 21 October and of his death. Despite the importance of the victory which removed the threat of invasion from England, the news of Nelson's death cast a gloom over London. 'He was,' Silliman observed, 'the very idol of this nation and the terror of its enemies.'[1]

On 29 October Silliman stayed overnight at Battersea Rise, the home of the banker and member of Parliament Henry Thornton, at Clapham then in the country outside London. Next morning at breakfast in the library he met William Wilberforce, who lived next door. Wilberforce and Thornton were then striving to abolish the trans-Atlantic slave trade, which they would succeed in outlawing by act of Parliament two years later. In the earnest evangelical atmosphere of the Thornton household Silliman found attitudes and values not unlike those of Yale College.

In late November Silliman left London for Edinburgh to attend lectures on various scientific subjects such as anatomy, chemistry, mineralogy, and medicine. In the chemistry lectures of Prof. Thomas Hope at the University of Edinburgh, Silliman heard the Huttonian theory of geology expounded, while in a private course of lectures on chemistry given by Mr. John Murray he had an opportunity to hear the opposing Wernerian theory defended. Silliman was thus a witness to the Huttonian-Wernerian debate at Edinburgh when it was at its height. On the whole Silliman leaned toward acceptance of the Wernerian theory. Soon after his arrival at Edinburgh he noted that Salisbury Craig bore 'a most striking resemblance' to East Rock at New Haven. On 8 January Silliman climbed Arthur's Seat to study its basaltic structure. The pillars of basalt, resembling those of the island of Staffa and the Giants Causeway in Ireland, formed well-defined prisms of six sides; 'three of the sides are visible,' Silliman noted, 'and three adhere to the mountain, as a pilaster to a building.'[2] Arthur's Seat, too, resembled the great rocks around New Haven, and Silliman became convinced that all of the ranges of pillared rocks in Connecticut, Massachusetts, and New Jersey were identical with the Scottish whinstone or traprock, which was basalt. One of the chief points of dispute between the Huttonians and Wernerians was over the origin of basalt. The Wernerians considered basalt a sedimentary rock formed by crystallization out of water, whereas the Huttonians thought that basalts had originated as vast sheets of molten lava.

At Edinburgh, Silliman found that scientific subjects were taught at a higher level and in a more thorough and polished manner than he had ever encountered before. Dr. Hope gave a complete course in chemistry in which he demonstrated, Silliman thought, 'an unrivalled example of neatness and beauty of experimental illustration.'[3]

Silliman shared a house with two fellow Americans, John Codman and John Gorham, both from Boston, Massachusetts, who were studying divinity. There were about twenty-five Americans studying medicine at Edinburgh, but most were from states south of New England. Silliman met and associated with many of the literary and scientific men who then made Edinburgh famous. At Dr. Hope's house Silliman met, but did not converse with, Dr. Robert Darwin, who would in three years' time become the father of Charles Robert Darwin, the future naturalist. Throughout his stay at Edinburgh, Silliman enjoyed the company of intelligent, congenial, and distinguished men. At one party Silliman met Archibald Constable and Alexander Gibson Hunter, who owned and published the astonishingly successful *Edinburgh Review*, a periodical which had first appeared only three years before. Silliman inquired into how the *Review* had been started and how it was managed, what salary the editor received, what was paid to writers, how large the circulation, and how issues were distributed. The remarkable feature of the *Edinburgh Review* was the generous scale on which it paid its authors, and the liveliness of its writing.

On 2 May 1806 Silliman sailed from Glasgow for New York, where he arrived on the 27th; and on Sunday afternoon, 1 June, he landed on the Long Wharf at New Haven in time to attend evening prayer at the Yale College chapel. Although only five weeks of the summer term remained, Silliman began to give a chemistry course to the Yale senior class. Thus began Silliman's teaching of science at Yale that continued each successive year until his retirement.

The years after 1806 were years of steady development for Silliman. His chemistry course was a regular part of the instruction for the senior class at Yale. In 1809 he married Harriet Trumbull, daughter of Jonathan Trumbull, governor of Connecticut, and the young couple moved to a house on Hillhouse Avenue that Silliman at first rented and later bought. In 1810 when Col. George Gibbs offered to deposit his mineralogical cabinet at Yale College, Silliman arranged to create a room in the college to contain it, and in 1815 he began to give lectures in mineralogy. In 1810 Silliman also played a leading role in the founding of the Medical Institution of Yale College, becoming professor of chemistry in the new medical school. In 1818 he founded the *American Journal of Science and the Arts* and alone edited it through the next twenty years.

In 1821 Silliman was given his first assistant, Sherlock J. Andrews, who had recently graduated from Union College at Schenectady, New York. Silliman was at that time beset by many sorrows and anxieties. In 1819 his eldest son, four years old, had died, followed two months later by his infant daughter. In 1820 and 1821 Silliman and his wife lost two more infant sons, each a few months after birth. The *American Journal of Science* proved a heavy and unceasing responsibility. In 1822 Silliman became ill with what was apparently a stomach ulcer, but by strict attention to diet he recovered gradually, and by 1823 was again in full health.

Sherlock Andrews assisted Silliman in the chemistry classes until 1823 when he left to become a lawyer. Silliman appointed his nephew, a Yale senior, for a year, followed by another young relative for a year, but neither wished to pursue careers in science. In 1826 Silliman appointed Charles Upham Shepard, a graduate of Amherst College, his assistant in chemistry. Shepard remained until 1831, but in 1828 Silliman also appointed Oliver Payson Hubbard, who remained Silliman's assistant until 1835 when he was succeeded by James Dwight Dana. In 1837 Dana in turn was succeeded by Silliman's own son Benjamin Silliman, Jr.

In 1834, at the request of several citizens of Hartford, Silliman gave a series of lectures on geology there during April and May. He proved extraordinarily successful as a public lecturer. He prepared his lectures very carefully and provided large drawings and samples of minerals. He was invited to lecture at Lowell, Massachusetts in September 1834. In February 1835, on the invitation of the Boston Society for Promoting Useful Knowledge, Silliman delivered his first lecture on geology at Boston in the Masonic Temple before an audience of 1,200 people. It was an enormous success and the Bostonians flocked to each of Silliman's subsequent lectures that lasted through March. In May 1835 Silliman gave a series of lectures at Salem, Massachusetts. From the first of June until nearly the end of August 1835 he was occupied with his geology course at Yale, but in September Silliman again spoke publicly, this time at Nantucket. In January 1836 Silliman lectured for the first time at New York City; in March and April 1836 he returned to Boston to present a second course and in May went to New York again. In January 1838 Silliman gave a double course on chemistry at New York, lectures of painful memory because he injured his foot severely during one lecture by dropping a six-pound weight on it.

In his first series of lectures at Boston in 1835, Silliman became well known and acquired many friends and acquaintances among Boston society. In June 1838 John Amory Lowell came to New Haven to consult Silliman about the organization of the Lowell Institute, newly established under the will of Mr. Lowell's cousin John Lowell, Jr. to provide scientific lectures for the public. Silliman agreed to give courses of Lowell lectures over a four-year period. In January 1840 Silliman delivered his first Lowell lecture series in the Odeon theatre at Boston on the subject of geology. Silliman also gave Lowell lectures in 1841, 1842, and 1843. In May 1843 Silliman lectured at Pittsburgh on geology and in March 1844 at Baltimore. Then in February 1845, Silliman, accompanied by Benjamin Silliman, Jr., went on an extended tour through the South. They traveled by railroad and steamboat first to Charleston, South Carolina where they saw Charles Upham Shepard and other scientists. Shepard was accustomed to spend several months of each winter at Charleston teaching chemistry at the South Carolina Medical College. From Charleston the Sillimans traveled across Georgia to Montgomery, Alabama and thence by steamboat down the Alabama River to Mobile where Silliman gave a series of lectures. After further courses of lectures at New Orleans and Natchez, Silliman and his son ascended the Mississippi and Ohio rivers by steamboat, marveling at the speed and comfort of their journey. In succeeding years Silliman lectured in many cities throughout New England, New York, and Pennsylvania. In 1852 he gave a series of lectures on geology at the Smithsonian Institution in Washington, D.C. and in 1855 at the age of seventy-five lectured at St. Louis. He found his voice no longer strong enough to fill a large hall and decided then not to attempt any more extended lecture tours. But he could not resist a few further engagements and as late as November 1857 gave a course at Buffalo, New York.

Silliman's career as a public lecturer on chemical and geological subjects, begun when he was already middle-aged, extended over a period of more than twenty years. His lectures made him a national scientific figure; they extended Silliman's reputation beyond the relatively small groups of students who attended his courses at Yale year after year, to the public at large. The success of the lectures rested both on a wonderfully effective exposition of scientific subjects—large drawings, many specimens of minerals and fossils, and brilliant chemical experiments that invariably worked—and on their character as lay sermons. In all natural phenomena Silliman saw the wisdom and goodness and the boundless providence of God everywhere manifested. Silliman saw himself as revealing one facet after another of the Almighty power present in the intricate and exact designs of a created universe. Such a message had a deep and broad appeal to the American public. Silliman aroused their curiosity, showed them natural wonders, entertained them with coruscating chemical demonstrations, and impressed them with his own kindly nature and sincere piety.

Benjamin Silliman was a large-minded and tolerant man. He encouraged, promoted, and assisted the efforts of John Pitkin Norton and Benjamin Silliman, Jr. to establish a scientific school at Yale in 1846. The gradual academic evolution of that school into the Yale Scientific School in 1854 and the Sheffield Scientific School in 1861 occurred with Silliman's unfailing encouragement, advice, and support. The beginning of graduate scientific education at the Sheffield Scientific School in 1861 was a culmination of Silliman's lifelong effort to establish both science teaching and scientific research in the United States.

In 1851 Benjamin Silliman went to Europe a second time. He was now seventy-one and left a widower by the death of Mrs. Silliman the year before; but he traveled with his old eagerness and enthusiasm, ready to compare the state of Europe in 1851 with what it had been in 1805. At London, Silliman visited the Great Exhibition, attended meetings of scientific societies, and for the first time met Gideon Mantell with whom he had corresponded on a basis of warm friendship for more than twenty years. From England, Silliman and his party made a truly grand tour through France, Italy, Sicily, Switzerland, Germany, and Belgium, returning finally to England to sail from Liverpool for New York. Once at home, he wrote and published a two-volume, detailed account of the journey.[4] On 17 September 1851, two days after his return to New Haven, Silliman married Mrs. Sarah Isabella Webb, an old friend of the family and a relative of his first wife, Harriet Trumbull.

In July 1853 as he approached his seventy-fourth birthday Benjamin Silliman formally retired from Yale. It was not a complete retirement; he remained a member of the Yale faculty as professor emeritus and was even asked to continue his lectures in mineralogy and geology until his son-in-law James Dwight Dana could assume responsibility for those subjects. Benjamin Silliman, Jr. succeeded his father in the chair of chemistry at Yale. Two years later, in 1855, Silliman, Jr. wrote a report on the composition of the rock oil of Venango County, Pennsylvania. By recognizing it to be a mixture of hydrocarbons that might be separated by fractional distillation, he launched the oil industry in the United States.

In retirement Benjamin Silliman was occupied pleasantly with putting his vast correspondence and various papers in order, and with his grandchildren. He also worked whenever possible to promote the development of Yale. In 1857 Silliman attempted to interest the financier George Peabody in the Yale Scientific School. This effort ultimately bore fruit in 1863 when Mr. Peabody decided to give $100,000 to Yale and asked that Professor Silliman act as one of his trustees. As the events that led to the Civil War gathered momentum, Silliman could not refrain from taking part. Although his father had owned slaves in Connecticut, Silliman had always opposed slavery. In February 1856 he was one of the speakers at a meeting in North

Church, New Haven, to raise money to buy rifles for the New England settlers in Kansas, and in July 1857 he joined in a private memorial to President Buchanan to protest the use of Federal troops to support the Southern faction in Kansas. When Buchanan publicized his reply, the New Haven group wrote a rejoinder and printed it with their original memorial and Buchanan's reply. Because Professor Silliman was better known than other signers of the memorial and rejoinder, he became the chief target for attack by newspapers sympathetic to the Buchanan administration, and the rejoinder became referred to as 'the Silliman letter.' Through the early years of the Civil War, Silliman anxiously watched the course of events, so frequently tragic and disastrous. In 1863 he was appointed a charter member of the newly formed National Academy of Sciences and attended the second meeting of the academy at New Haven in August 1864. On 4 November 1864, the day after attending a meeting to hear reports of the work of the Sanitary Commission in caring for sick and wounded soldiers, Silliman took ill. Three weeks later on Thanksgiving morning, 24 November 1864, he died.

NOTES

[1] Silliman, *Travels*, II, 200.
[2] *Ibid.*, II, 303.
[3] *Ibid.*, II, 312.
[4] Silliman, *Visit to Europe*.

Protestantism, Science, and American Enterprise: Benjamin Silliman's Moral Universe

JOHN C. GREENE

BENJAMIN SILLIMAN did not choose science for his life's work. He was chosen for science by his revered teacher Timothy Dwight, president of Yale College from 1795 to 1817, resolute foe of 'infidelity' in all its forms, and staunch advocate of the view that science, far from being the enemy of the Christian religion, was its natural ally. During his tenure as tutor at Yale, Dwight had worked through Newton's *Principia* three times, ruining his eyes and health by prolonged study and fasting. Elected president of Yale at a time when 'infidelity' was widespread on American campuses, he resolved to meet squarely the Enlightenment's challenge to Christian faith by introducing chemistry and natural history into the curriculum and placing them in the care of one whom he himself had imbued with sound Christian understanding.

Such a one was Benjamin Silliman, son of Gen. Gold Selleck Silliman, lawyer, Revolutionary War hero, and descendant of a long line of pious Puritans. 'Sober Ben' young Silliman was called when he began his studies at Yale in 1792. Three years later, when Timothy Dwight took charge of the college, delivering a full course of sermons on Christian doctrine to the junior and senior classes annually, he found an attentive and admiring auditor in the serious young man from Fairfield.

> He is truly a great man [Silliman wrote in his diary], and it is very rare that so many excellent natural and acquired endowments are to be found in one person. When I hear him speak, it makes me feel like a very insignificant being, and almost prompts me to despair; but I am reencouraged when I reflect that he was once as ignorant as myself, and that learning is only to be acquired by long and assiduous application.

At a time when physical science had not yet captured the popular imagination, Dwight 'saw with a telescopic view both its intrinsic importance and its practical relations to the wants of man and to the progress of society.'[1]

It was Timothy Dwight who, having molded Silliman's ideas and ideals by the powerful influence of his personality and preaching, now

11

enlisted his talents in the cause of science. Silliman had displayed no particular enthusiasm for science during his studies at Yale. Two years after graduation he could find in himself 'no propensity . . . stronger than a wish to be highly *respectable* and *respected*' in the legal profession, in which his father and grandfather had distinguished themselves. But Dwight had other plans for him. On a July morning in 1801, during a chance encounter on the college grounds, Dwight astonished Silliman by offering him the newly established professorship of chemistry and natural history at Yale.

> In the profession which I proffer to you [Dwight urged] there will be no rival here. The field will be all your own. The study will be full of interest and gratification, and the presentation which you will be able to make of it to the college classes and the public will afford much instruction and delight. Our country, as regards the physical sciences, is rich in unexplored treasures, and by aiding in their development you will perform an important public service, and connect your name with the rising reputation of our native land.[2]

Although Silliman did not mention it in his report of this conversation, one wonders whether President Dwight may not also have alluded to the opportunity Silliman would have to display the harmony of science and religion—an undertaking of the greatest importance in Dwight's estimation, and one for which Silliman, just then undergoing full conversion to the Christian faith, would be especially well fitted. Whether uttered or not, such a thought must surely have been in Dwight's mind.

The story of Silliman's subsequent career—his studies in Philadelphia, London, and Edinburgh, his brilliant success as a teacher and promoter of the sciences at Yale, his outstanding contribution as founder and editor of the *American Journal of Science*, his influence as a public lecturer on chemistry and geology, his practical services as consulting chemist and geologist, and his role in helping to organize the scientific community in the United States—all this has been narrated elsewhere. The aim of the present essay will be to investigate his intellectual and moral universe to discover the controlling ideas and sentiments that shaped his words and actions in the many fields of endeavor to which he applied his talents. Every noble and useful life springs from some enduring vision of the world and man's place in it, from an ideal of individual and social existence. In Silliman's mind the driving force, apart from the normal human aspiration to succeed in one's calling and win the respect and admiration of one's fellow human beings, was a profound acceptance of the Christian view of nature, man, and society which had been instilled in him in childhood and given intellectual form and content by the sermons of Timothy Dwight.

The clearest exposition of Silliman's conception of science and its place in the general scheme of things is to be found in the introductory lecture to his course in chemistry at Yale, published in 1828 at the request of his students. After stating that man was distinguished from 'the various orders of inferior animals' by his God-given capacity for knowledge, Silliman undertook to survey the domain of human knowledge. He began with moral science, 'which informs us of our relation to the Creator, and to each other.' But moral science was dependent upon religion, which in turn was based on God's revelation of Himself in the Bible as its 'principal, and only infallible source,' although some light on religion and morality could be derived from 'nature justly viewed.' 'These few [Biblical] allusions alone,' Silliman declared, 'contain our justification for studying the works of the Creator, which are pronounced to be *very good*; and they repress our pride and exclude every approach of atheism, by informing us whence the creation arose, and what will be its final catastrophe.'[3]

Passing over language, 'one of the most important gifts of God to man,' rhetoric, 'the accurate, elegant and energetic exhibition, of the thoughts of the mind,' and logic, 'the art of reasoning,' Silliman came next to metaphysics, 'the science which treats of the general affections of being; of the first principles of our knowledge and of our universal ideas.' Conceding that this subject had been greatly abused, he insisted nevertheless that every science had its own metaphysics, 'and to the eye of God, who perfectly and intuitively comprehends the whole, there is no where either obscurity or inconsistency, but all is harmonious and excellent, in every department of knowledge, and in every province of the immense creation, of mind and matter.' Referring again to God the Creator toward the end of his lecture, he acknowledged but three sources of information about reality—'His works, His ways, and His word.' Correctly understood, these formed a single harmonious system, the discovery and admiration of which was the object of human understanding. 'Knowledge,' Silliman told his pupils, 'is nothing but the just and full comprehension of the real nature of things, physical, intellectual, and moral; it is coextensive with the universe of being, both material and spiritual; it reaches back to the dawn of time, and forward to its consummation; nay, it is coeval with eternity, and is inseparable from the incomprehensible existence of Jehovah. Only one mind, therefore, intuitively embraces the whole.'[4]

On these premises, it was clear to Silliman that science, or
knowledge of the natural world, was valuable both as an intellectual
discipline leading man to a knowledge of his Creator through the study
of His works and as a God-given means whereby man could provide for
his physical needs. Every branch of science had its related arts which
could be improved and perfected by the application of scientific
principles. 'Chemistry,' he explained, 'is distinguished as *an art* or a
collection of arts, from *chemistry* as a science; the former is empirical,
the latter is guided by established principles.'

> The reason why *art* and *science* mutually aid each other is, that art
> furnishes hands and science eyes; science without art is inefficient, art
> without science is blind.
>   The chemist must understand the *principles* of the chemical arts, and
> the more of the practice the better.
>   Chemical artists should understand the science, at least of their own
> arts, and practical knowledge is of course indispensable.[5]

In Silliman's view, chemistry was at one and the same time 'a
branch of general Philosophy,' 'a school for the chemical arts and for
many of those of domestic economy,' and 'an important auxiliary to
the profession of medicine and to pharmacy.' But it was not to be
valued only for its utility: 'It would now be as disreputable for any
person, claiming to have received a liberal education, or to possess
liberal knowledge, to be ignorant of the great principles and of the
leading facts of chemical as of mechanical philosophy.' Medicine,
likewise, was not simply a practical art. Every medical student—
Silliman had many of them—should study the sciences and should
aspire to add something to the body of scientific knowledge, thereby
becoming 'entitled to a distinguished rank among philosophers.'

For Silliman science was not just an intellectual exercise or an
instrument for bending nature to the satisfaction of human needs. It
was at the same time a quest for insight into the harmony of the cosmos
and the character of its Creator. Moral beings, declared Silliman,
'cannot cultivate even physical science, without imparting to their
labors a moral bearing; . . . we are responsible for the use which we
make of natural science.'

In keeping with these general views, Silliman tried to maintain a
balance between the intellectual, moral, religious, and utilitarian
aspects of science in all his undertakings—as teacher, author, editor,
public lecturer, consulting chemist and geologist, and educational
statesman. In his academic lectures, his one time assistant Charles
Upham Shepard recalled that Silliman 'greatly increased the interest of

his subject by reference to useful applications, and by anticipations of others in the immediate future.'

> At that early day [wrote Shepard] . . . steam was but half applied. Houses and streets were lighted, only prospectively, by gas. Little was known of magnetism beyond the directive power of the needle, or of electricity except in the electric machine and the lightning rod, so that when it was foretold that these two great powers were soon to rival heat itself in their beneficent uses, the prediction seemed to belong more to the imagination than to science; and yet we of today [1885] witness its near fulfillment.

Yet, as always, Silliman placed these actual and prospective triumphs of applied science in a Christian context. 'There was reference also to something higher and more excellent,' Shepard recalled. 'The Divine Power . . . was often acknowledged in fitting expressions. . . .'[6]

The same solicitude to put science in proper perspective was evident in the textbooks Silliman wrote or edited for class use. In the introduction to his *Elements of Chemistry in the Order of the Lectures Given in Yale College* (1830-31) Silliman reproduced much of the 'Introductory Lecture' already described. The student of chemistry, he added,

> finds, everywhere, innumerable applications of his knowledge to purposes of practical utility, to those of domestic life, to the arts which enrich and adorn society, and to the illustration of the wisdom, power and goodness of that great being, whose pleasure called the physical universe into existence and constantly sustains it in order and beauty.
>
> Literature adorns and illustrates science, adding much to its attractions, and to the method, perspicuity, and effect of its communications. It cannot be entirely neglected, by any one who would claim an elevated rank in physical science.

As to scientific method, Silliman adopted Newton's 'rules of philosophising,' adding a few of his own:

> The moral effect of physical study upon every mind which has been correctly disciplined, is altogether happy, and augments the vigor of every proper feeling. It is not, however, to be denied, that an opposite effect is sometimes produced upon certain minds; but this is the fault of the individual and not of the study. . . .
>
> The greatest mental power and the longest life, joined with the greatest industry, can enable man to compass only a small part of universal knowledge.[7]

The main body of the text, comprising two substantial volumes profusely illustrated with diagrams and descriptions of experiments from Robert Hare's *Compendium of Chemistry*, exhibited Silliman's powers of organization and exposition and his broad view of chemistry in relation to natural philosophy. A modern historian of chemistry, Aaron J. Ihde, evaluates Silliman's *Elements* as follows:

> ... I am very favorably impressed by the book. It must, of course, be reviewed in the context of the times; it stands up very well against equivalent textbooks coming out of England, France, and Germany. The treatment is entirely descriptive in character, primarily because there is no theory of consequence at the time. The discussion of light, heat, and attraction is up-to-date and reflects the points of view which are character-istic of the paradigms of the times. The treatment of the various elements is exceedingly thorough. ... It is obvious ... that although the United States was outside the mainstream of chemical activities, Silliman had gone to great pains to keep abreast of developments in Europe. He discusses the experiments of the foremost chemists and is obviously a good enough chemist to understand these experiments and their significance. The two volumes contain experimental directions for carrying out student experiments, and these directions are well conceived.[8]

In the field of geology, Silliman never wrote a textbook, preferring to use Robert Bakewell's *Introduction to Geology* with an appendix of his own. In the first American edition of Bakewell (1829), Silliman was still a convinced Wernerian, attributing to aqueous agency many phenomena which most geologists ascribed to the effects of heat and pressure. By 1839, however, he had altered his views in the light of the publications of Lyell, Scrope, Daubeny, and others—'I have been for a series of years in a condition to do full justice to the internal agency of fire, as my various classes in the university and elsewhere can attest.'[9]

The chief purpose of Silliman's appendix to the American editions, however, was to vindicate geology from the charge of being hostile to the claims and interests of revealed religion. Declaring his firm adherence to 'the Baconian and Newtonian mode of reasoning on natural phenomena,' he was concerned nevertheless, like Newton, to display 'their ultimate connexion with the Creator and Governor of the universe' and their compatibility with Scripture. In 1829 he took the position that 'every great feature in the structure of the planet corre-sponds with the *order of the events* narrated in sacred history' and that physical effects of the biblical Deluge were identifiable on the surface of the earth.

A decade later, however, he was prepared to concede that the correspondence between the paleontological record and the events described in Genesis was only approximate and that 'amidst the vast exuberance of diluvial remains, it is impossible to appropriate to the general deluge, those that belong to it, rather than to more local debacles, and to those of a different era.' The main point of concern, he insisted, was the vast amount of time required to produce the present appearances on the earth's surface by the operation of everyday processes of matter in motion. By interpreting the biblical word for *day* to mean a period of indefinite length, one could provide the necessary amount of time within the scriptural framework. Once this was done, the detailed reconciliation of geological discoveries with the sacred history could safely be left to future investigation.

'No geologist, at the present day,' Silliman declared, 'erects any system upon the basis of Scripture history, or any other history.' But there was nothing to prevent the geologist from noting the coincidences between the findings of science and the events narrated in the Bible. 'This he will do merely on the ground of historical and geological coincidence, and without drawing for the support of his scientific views upon any portion of his moral feeling, towards a work which, as an individual, he may revere as a communication from his Maker, for purposes far more important than the establishment of physical truth.' [10]

Silliman's concern to maintain a balanced view of the role of science in human civilization was equally evident in his conduct of the journal he founded and edited for more than a quarter of a century, *The American Journal of Science*. Its early title, *The American Journal of Science and the Arts*, is indicative of the scope and purpose of the journal as initially conceived by Silliman. 'This Journal,' Silliman announced in his 'Plan of the Work' in the first volume, 'is intended to embrace the circle of the PHYSICAL SCIENCES, with their application to the Arts, and to every useful purpose. While SCIENCE will be cherished for its own sake, and with a due respect for its own *inherent* dignity; it will also be employed as the handmaid to the Arts.' Silliman mentioned here agriculture, manufactures (both mechanical and chemical), and domestic economy. He also invited communications on music, sculpture, engraving, painting, and, more generally, on the fine and liberal as well as the useful arts.

In the end, Silliman had to give up the idea of including the fine arts within the purview of his journal, but he continued to solicit articles on improvements in the practical arts, especially improvements involving applications of the principles of science. In the preface to the second volume he stressed that his journal was national, not local, in its coverage and that its 'leading object' was 'to advance the interests of this rising empire, by exciting and concentrating original American effort, both in the sciences, and in the arts.' He appealed to his fellow countrymen to support an enterprise designed to advance the wealth and power, the honor and dignity, of 'the vast American Republic, with ten millions of inhabitants, with wealth scarcely surpassed by that of the most favoured nations, and with immensely diversified interests, growing out of those physical resources, which the bounty of God has given us.'[11]

In accord with these aims, Silliman admitted to his *Journal* articles on the use of tar and steam as fuel, American porcelain clays, a new inflammable air lamp, scientifically based improvements in the construction of the printing press, Jacob Perkins's method of engraving upon steel, Ithiel Town's new idea for the design of bridges, Daguerre's technique of fixing photographic images, Morse's telegraph, the invention of electroplating, W. R. Johnson's experiments for the U.S. Navy on the heating power of various types of coal, Thomas Davenport's electromagnetic machine, and many other practical improvements. At the same time, Silliman kept in touch with the practical world of invention and business enterprise. He was a lifelong friend of Eli Whitney, who graduated from Yale in the year that Silliman entered college and who later invited Silliman to join him on a tour of Europe for the purpose of securing patents on his cotton gin. Although Silliman did not accept the invitation, the two men became good friends. In 1808 Silliman asked Whitney to devise a method of casting tin tubes to be used for transmitting soda water (which was just beginning to be known in America).

Silliman also made friends with Charles Goodyear and gave him much-needed encouragement in his experiments with rubber.

> One day I called on him at his humble cottage on Washington hill . . . and found him making some of his preparations over the stove, while some of his family were sick. He told me afterwards that my visit encouraged him, and that, as I left the door, I told him to persevere, that something important would come of his researches, and that when he should be ready, I would make a noise about it, as I did in my lectures in Yale College and by my influence.[12]

Thomas Davenport, too, received encouragement when he came to New Haven to show Silliman his electromagnetic machine. The result was a handsome notice of this machine, as well as of another constructed by Israel Slade of Troy, New York, in the *American Journal of Science* in 1837. The main difference between the two machines was that Davenport's used only electromagnets, whereas Slade's employed permanent magnets as well. Tremendously impressed by Davenport's machine, Silliman urged that these investigations should be 'prosecuted with zeal, *aided by correct scientific knowledge,* by *mechanical skill,* and by *ample funds.*' He told the readers of his *Journal* that

> Science has thus, most unexpectedly, placed in our hands a new power of great but unknown energy. . . . Nothing since the discovery of gravitation and of the structure of the celestial systems, is so wonderful as the power evolved by galvanism. . . . It may therefore be reasonably hoped, that science and art, the handmaids of discovery, will both receive from this interesting research, a liberal reward.[13]

While he celebrated the triumphs of applied science in his *Journal,* Silliman did not lose sight of the religious and moral aspects. In a letter to Prof. Parker Cleaveland of Bowdoin College in 1817 outlining his plans for the *Journal,* Silliman had raised the question: 'Would our infidels and light minded folk bear to have geology made to illustrate the truth of the Mosaic history of which I am fully persuaded it demonstrates the truth?'[14] As editor of the *American Journal of Science,* however, Silliman did not belabor the subject of science and religion. There were occasional notices of the founding and activities of Bible and tract societies, and in 1834 Silliman reprinted lengthy excerpts from an article in the *Edinburgh New Philosophical Journal* under the title 'Remarks on the Connection Between the Mosaic History of the Creation and the Discoveries of Geology, Occasioned by the Lectures of Baron Cuvier on the History of the Natural Sciences,' including a 'Table of Coincidences Between the Order of Events as Described in Genesis, and That Unfolded by Geological Investigation.' For the most part, however, he was content to let science speak for itself with only an occasional reminder that 'science is only embodied and systematized truth, and . . . *it tells the thoughts of God.*'

In his activities as a consulting chemist and geologist—a new role for the American scientist—Silliman took a broad and balanced view of his opportunities and duties, combining a patriotic enthusiasm for American economic development with a strong conviction of the moral responsibility of business entrepreneurs. As a chemist he was called upon by the United States government to prepare a report on the cultivation of sugar cane and the refining of sugar, and the Connecticut River Steam Boat Company hired him to investigate the causes of the explosion which shattered the steamboat *New England* in October 1833.

But his chief role as a consultant was in connection with mining ventures. As early as 1809 Silliman was asked by a group of Boston merchants to assess the mineral potential of a lead mine in Northampton, Massachusetts. In the 1830s he was hired successively by groups of investors interested in mineral lands in the Wyoming and Lackawanna valleys of Pennsylvania, in gold mining properties in Goochland, Culpeper, Louisa, and Fauquier counties in Virginia, and in coal and iron lands in western Maryland. His reports, published for publicity purposes by the companies involved and republished in part by Silliman in the *American Journal of Science,* throw considerable light on the beginnings of scientific consulting in the United States. Assisted at various times and in various ways by his son, by Professors Edward Hitchcock and Charles Upham Shepard of Amherst College, and by George Jones, senior tutor at Yale, Silliman took note not merely of the geology and mineralogy of the regions he surveyed but also of the availability of transportation, waterpower for operating machinery, and timber for fuel, as well as problems of mine drainage, optimum routes for building rail connections to mine properties, and prospects for realizing a profit on investments in these lands. He was, in short, a consulting economist and engineer as well as chemist and geologist.

Carried away with the prospects for American economic development, Silliman sometimes displayed a patriotic enthusiasm for individual and corporate enterprise worthy of a modern chamber of commerce. Of the Wyoming Valley in Pennsylvania he wrote:

> The noble mine, railway and canal, of the Delaware and Hudson company, show what can be done, by the resources, enterprise and perseverance of an association of individuals; and it cannot be doubted that the two most opulent and powerful States in the Union, having already led the way . . . in the great field of internal improvement, will continue to consult the high interests of their citizens, by completing all the communications and especially the northern ones, with this valley. . . . The importance of the coal beds will justify and require a canal on each side of the river, and numerous rail ways leading from different mines. We may expect soon to see this noble valley become a great thorough fare of travelling and of business, and a seat of numerous manufactures, for which its great fertility, its vast magazines of fuel, its fine water powers, and its excellent population, give it rare advantages.[15]

Concerning the Howell lands in western Maryland, Silliman was even more ecstatic:

> The inexhaustible supplies of coal and iron ores, both of the best quality, the coal being particularly adapted by its peculiarities for the successful manufacture of iron in its various forms; the limestone, common and

hydraulic; the fireclays, the sandstones, and millstonegrit; the forests; the agricultural productions; the sheep and cattle, with abundant hay and pastorage for their support; the fine climate; the central position in relation to the ancient east, and the young and rising west; the great national road intersecting the region; the grand canal, soon to give a permanent and sufficient outlet for these hitherto sealed treasures; and an unlimited demand arising from the boundless wants of our great and rapidly growing country, calling not only for fuel and iron, but for every product which can be manufactured by human skill and industry, managed by the dense population that will hereafter occupy this remarkable region; all these facts and circumstances afford the strongest assurance that those who, with proper resources, with skill and judgment, with integrity and perseverance, engage in the great enterprises which the resources of the Frostburgh region so decidedly encourage, and are able so fully to sustain, will not be disappointed, but will reap a rich reward, and contribute efficiently to the permanent honour and prosperity of their country, and to the good of mankind.[16]

In Silliman's mind the fortunate proximity of argillaceous iron ores to vast coal deposits was no accident. It seemed rather to indicate 'a wise and benevolent design in the Author of nature, since nothing can be more happy than to find the most important of all the metals in the same mines with the fuel ready for working it. . . .'

At the same time, however, that Silliman called attention to the bountiful resources Providence had prepared for economic development by American enterprise, he took pains to make clear that both Providence and patriotism forbade the buying and selling of mineral lands for speculative profit. Reporting to the Richmond Mining Company in 1836 at the height of the gold mining boom in Virginia and of the speculative mania that was to produce the Panic of 1837, Silliman warned his employers against the 'spirit of speculation.'

The speculator who buys merely that he may sell again is, too frequently, imperfectly informed in the facts, and reckless also of the consequences in regard to those who may succeed him in his obligations; frequent gains from sales of stock are reported from day to day; the property rapidly changes hands; the public mind being morbidly excited, is of course blinded, and at no distant period, accumulated ruin falls heavily upon the last in the train. This is exactly the opposite of the mental sobriety and moral rectitude which ought to govern men in all concerns, and especially in such transactions as these; it is not too much to say, that no man should either buy or sell a mining interest, unless he can, in honor and conscience, declare that he believes it can be profitably carried on. . . .[17]

In the mind of this Christian professor of science in mid-nineteenth century New England, piety, patriotism, science, practical invention, and business enterprise were welded together in a fervent vision of the noble destiny prepared by God for the inhabitants of a favored land, if only they would pursue that destiny in obedience to God's revelation in the Bible of His purpose for man. One wonders what Silliman would say if he could view the state of his beloved country after a century and a half of progress in science, technology, and business enterprise, if not in mental sobriety and moral rectitude.

On the public lecture platform Silliman found even greater opportunity to present science in all its aspects—intellectual, practical, moral, and religious. The number of his auditors reached into the thousands. In Boston he attracted 'four times a week 3,000 people in two divisions of 1500 each,' drawn from all classes of society. In Lowell the female factory workers turned out to hear him in large numbers. In Hartford he drew an audience of 300 to 400, in Nantucket about the same number, in New York nearly a thousand, in Pittsburgh and Baltimore about 600, in Mobile 250, in New Orleans 500, in Natchez 120. He also lectured successfully in Cincinnati, St. Louis, Philadelphia, Reading, Washington, and Brooklyn. Chemistry and geology and their technological applications and religious and moral implications were matters of great public interest, and Silliman was exactly the man to treat these subjects in a manner that was intellectually fascinating and psychologically reassuring. His teaching at Yale had taught him the utility of well-performed experiments to fix the attention of an audience, 'it being . . . an absolute rule, that nothing capable of visual representation should be omitted.' His assistant Charles Upham Shepard recalled:

> During the lecture hour there was no lull or intermission; all was rapid movement, a constant appeal to the delighted senses. Here were broad irradiations of emerald phosphoresence, there the vivid spangles of burning iron, or the blinding effulgence of the compound blow-pipe, or the galvanic deflagrator. Strange sounds saluted the ear, from the singing hydrogen tube, the crackling decrepitation up to the loud explosions of mingled gases and detonating fulminates. As forms of matter once regarded simple were torn into their elements, or these again compounded in manifold ways, a very kaleidoscope of changes came into view, of which the greatest was the transformation of the whole seeming phantasy into science, through the lucid rationale of the gifted lecturer.[18]

The demonstrations which amazed and delighted the Yale undergraduates were equally effective with audiences in Boston, Salem, and

Nantucket. 'The people are astonished to see intense ignition coming out of cold fluids and the rocks themselves melting under a stream of burning gases,' Silliman noted in his private journal. Few other lecturers could hold an audience spellbound for an hour and a half to two hours. 'In person,' reported the *New York Tribune*, 'Professor Silliman is tall, stoutly built, and has a highly intellectual and thoughtful countenance. His delivery is extremely rapid, more so than any other lecturer we have heard; he seems to speak from the fullest knowledge of his subject and with an energy and enthusiasm which frequently carry him from the main topic into collateral, though most interesting, discussions.' A more rough and ready evaluation of his performance was provided by two auditors whom Silliman overheard in the following dialogue: 'He is a smart old fellow,' said one man. 'Yes, he is a real steam boat,' replied the other.

The effectiveness of his presentation was but one factor in Silliman's success. Equally important was his reiterated assurance that science and religion were in perfect harmony. Again and again, as in New York, he declared in these or similar words:

> Our histories may lie. . . . But the rocks cannot lie. . . . Nor need the religious fear any subversion of their faith, nor infidels hope for any support from geology; as the slanderers of the science falsely declare. All the objects of geology aim at truth; and among the many distinguished geologists I have known, I have found but one or two infidels. Truth is always truth, and no one truth . . . can ever be in conflict with any others.[19]

Or, at Pittsburgh:

> The book of Genesis is not a scientific treatise . . . , & must not be so considered. Yet, though I look not for entire agreement . . . , in the integrity of an honest man, I declare, that I know of no conflict between them [geology and the Bible]. True science is fitted to teach us how the laws of nature are employed to produce the happy issues which everywhere present themselves to our admiring contemplation. . . . Except the soul of man, everything created is progressive.[20]

These assurances, coming from a man of commanding presence, high social prestige, and solid scientific reputation, did as much to produce near-veneration in Silliman's audiences as did his skill and clarity in presenting the discoveries of chemistry and geology. The *Boston Transcript* reported:

> Admiring as we do the perfection of science exhibited continually by the lecturer . . . , we have yet a higher love and reverence for that beautiful exhibition of divine truth to which Mr. Silliman constantly alludes, as

seen in the wonderful works which he has successfully presented as designed by the Almighty power, and made known to man by human intelligence. This is the source of our respect for this accomplished Professor, in comparison with which our admiration for his scientific attainments sinks into insignificance.[21]

Silliman himself placed no less a value on this aspect of his success as a public lecturer and 'apostle of Geology.' Grateful as he was for the financial remuneration—over $22,000 in total—which these lectures brought him and for 'the satisfying assurance that I have popularized science,' he was even more grateful for the opportunity they gave him to illustrate the 'theology of nature.' 'For my signal success I have devoutly thanked my Maker & if there was any honor I gave it all to him, regarding myself as only the humble exponent of his laws in a portion of his ways.'[22] As to the total effect of Silliman's lectures both at Yale and before the general public, we have the testimony of no less reliable an observer than Sir Charles Lyell, who wrote to Silliman in 1842:

> Now that I have travelled from Niagara to Georgia, and have met a great number of your countrymen on the Continent of Europe, and heard the manner in which they ascribe the taste they have for science to your tuition, I may congratulate you, for I never heard as many of the rising generation in England refer as often to any one individual teacher as having given a direction to their taste.[23]

Compared with the foregoing contributions to the development of American science, Silliman's additions to scientific knowledge itself were very modest. His geological publications were confined to descriptive accounts of parts of Connecticut and such out-of-state regions as he visited in the course of business or pleasure. Concerning these publications a modern geologist, Janet Aitken, has written:

> ... in geology he was essentially a mineralogist-petrographer with a strong focus on igneous rock, basalts in particular. . . . The most solid parts of his papers are almost invariably mineralogical or petrographical in nature. . . . His contributions to the professional literature were minimal compared to those of [Charles T.] Jackson in northern New England, those of [Edward] Hitchock in Massachusetts, or more widely, those of Maclure, Dana or Eaton. Quite possibly his professorial and editorial duties precluded a very substantial bibliography in this area. In the main he seems to have functioned as an instigator, inspiring and urging others to provide the details that would embellish and refine his broad-brush geological portraits.[24]

On the experimental side, Silliman's research efforts were devoted chiefly to the fusion of refractory substances with the aid of the oxyhydrogen blowpipe and the deflagrator, both invented by his good friend Robert Hare. Experiments of this kind were standard fare in his courses, and they did much to prove that almost any substance is fusible if sufficient heat is applied to it. In his experiments on the fusion of carbon, he noted the transfer of volatilized carbon from the positive electrode to the negative pole. Of all his publications, his first, the Silliman-Kingsley account of the Weston meteor in 1809, attracted more attention internationally than any other.[25]

That these contributions to the literature of science were of minimal importance to the progress of chemistry, mineralogy, and geology Silliman himself would have been the first to concede. But he would not have been greatly disturbed by the admission. For he knew that through his teaching, his lecturing, his textbook, his editorship of the *American Journal of Science*, his part in organizing the American Geological Society and the American Association of Geologists, and his support of graduate education in science at Yale he had done as much to advance the cause of science in his native country as any American. For him science was not a passion, a burning desire to discover the hidden secrets of nature, to find out why things are as they are, to reduce the welter of phenomena to mathematical rule. The late nineteenth-century conception of science as the *summum bonum*, as a quest for natural knowledge regardless of its practical utility and its bearing on morality and religion (or, alternatively, as the guarantor of human progress and the only avenue to knowledge of any kind) would have struck him as irrational and impious. To him natural science was but one of many fields of human activity, but one part of universal knowledge, but one gift of the Creator, who would hold mankind responsible for its proper use. Writing the closing paragraphs of his 'Reminiscences' at the age of eighty-two, he reflected:

> . . . I can truly declare, that in the study and exhibition of science to my pupils and fellow-men, I have never forgotten to give all the honor and glory to the infinite Creator,—happy if I might be the honored interpreter of a portion of His works, and of the beautiful structure and beneficent laws discovered therein by the labors of many illustrious predecessors. For this I claim no merit. It is the result to which right reason and sound philosophy, as well as religion, would naturally lead.[26]

To the twentieth-century mind, obsessed by fears of nuclear destruction and environmental pollution, Silliman's simple faith in the progressive tendency of science, technology, and business enterprise regulated by Protestant piety and biblically-based morality seems hopelessly naive in the light of subsequent events. But his resolute effort to see human life and the place of science in it steadily and to see it whole should commend itself to all who value right reason and sound philosophy, to say nothing of religion.

NOTES

[1] Quoted in Fulton and Thomson, *Silliman*, p. 13.

[2] Quoted from Silliman's manuscript 'Reminiscences,' in Fisher, *Silliman*, I, 93.

[3] Silliman, *Introductory Lecture*, p. 7.

[4] *Ibid.*, p. 47.

[5] *Ibid.*, p. 37.

[6] Charles U. Shepard, 'Address of Presentation,' in *Memorial Addresses*, p. 10.

[7] Silliman, *Elements of Chemistry*, I, 174.

[8] Letter from Prof. Aaron J. Ihde to the author, 24 February 1971. I am grateful to Professor Ihde for permission to quote this letter.

[9] Silliman, 'Philosophy of Geology,' p. 463.

[10] *Ibid.*, pp. 573, 575.

[11] *Am. J. Sci.*, 1820, 2, Preface. See also Preface, vol. 1.

[12] Quoted in Fisher, *Silliman*, II, 280–281. Silliman's relations with Eli Whitney are described in his 'Reminiscences of the Late Mr. Whitney, Inventor of the Cotton Gin,' *Am. J. Sci.*, 1832, 21, 255–264.

[13] [Silliman], 'Notice of the Electro-Magnetic Machine of Mr. Thomas Davenport of Brandon, near Rutland, Vermont,' *Am. J. Sci.*, 1837, 32, appendix to no. 1, p. 7.

[14] Silliman to Cleaveland, 6 October 1817, Cleaveland Correspondence.

[15] Silliman, *Report on the Coal Formation of the Valleys of Wyoming and Lacka-wanna*, p. 10; republished in part in the *Am. J. Sci.*, 1830, 18, 308–328.

[16] Silliman and Silliman, Jr., *Extracts From A Report Made to the New York and Maryland Coal & Iron Company*, pp. 36–37.

[17] Silliman, *To the President and Directors of the Richmond Mining Company*, pp. 12–13; reprinted in *Am. J. Sci.*, 1837, 32, 98–130. This pamphlet may be seen at the Beinecke Library, Yale University. Other mining reports by Silliman may be found in the Blake Family Papers.

[18] Shepard (n. 6), pp. 9–10.

[19] Clipping from *New York Tribune*, 13 February 1842, in vol. 6 of Silliman, 'Reminiscences', Silliman Family Papers.

[20] Silliman, *Lectures on Geology*, p. 34.

[21] Quoted from the *Boston Transcript*, 30 March 1843, in Fisher, *Silliman*, I, 398.

[22] Silliman, 'Reminiscences,' VII, 154, Silliman Family Papers.

[23] Charles Lyell to Silliman, 4 April 1842, quoted in Fisher, *Silliman*, II, 163–164.

[24] Communication from Prof. Janet Aitken, Emeritus Professor of Geology, University of Connecticut, quoted with the kind permission of Professor Aitken.

[25] Silliman's contributions to mineralogy, including his chemical analysis of the Weston meteor, are discussed in the forthcoming work by Greene and Burke, *Science of Minerals in the Age of Jefferson.*

[26] Quoted in Fisher, *Silliman*, II, 23.

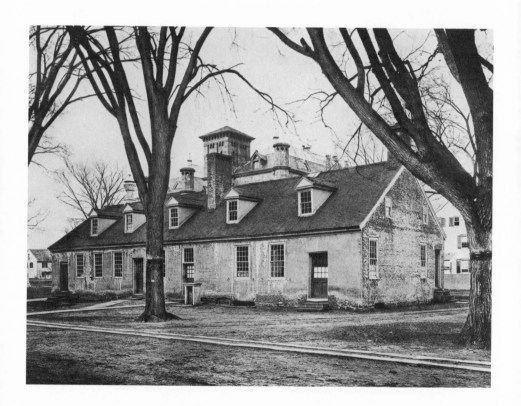

Chemistry laboratory used by Benjamin Silliman.

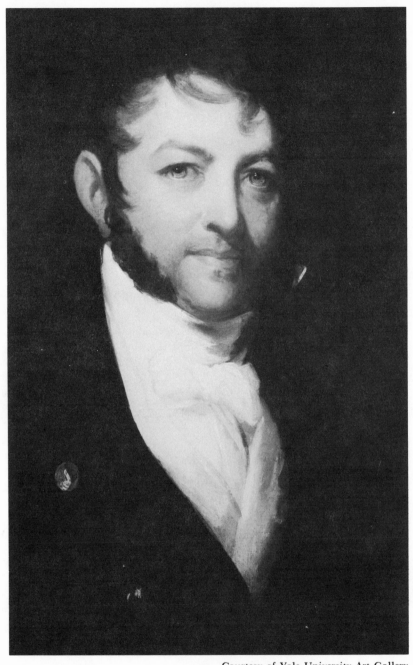

*Colonel George Gibbs, about 1830. Artist unknown,
copy after Gilbert Stuart.*

Colonel George Gibbs

STEPHEN DOW BECKHAM

THE SETTING was Fulton's packet steamer scudding from port to port on Long Island Sound. The time was November 1817. Prof. Benjamin Silliman of Yale University and Col. George Gibbs of Sunswick Farms, Astoria, New York were deep in conversation. Drawn together more than a decade earlier by mutual interests in science, the two friends were discussing the condition of American opportunities in research and publication. As Silliman later recalled, Gibbs suddenly pressed the subject of a new scientific journal—one that Silliman should edit. The proposal, enthusiastically embraced by the Yale professor, led in July 1818, to the first issue of the *American Journal of Science and the Arts*, or, as it was more popularly known through much of the nineteenth century, Silliman's *Journal*.[1]

Fortune and friendship were the ingredients that drew Gibbs and Silliman together that day in 1817 on Long Island Sound. The latter element, friendship, was a mutual appreciation for geology and the mysteries of nature. The former element, fortune, was largely Gibbs's monopoly, for his life was one of luck and wealth. He had riches in family, friends, and money.

Col. George Gibbs, the third of his lineage in America to bear the name, was born 7 January 1776, at Newport, Rhode Island. His great grandfather, James Gibbs, had emigrated to the colony about 1670 from England. James and his son George were farmers. It was with the second George Gibbs, born in 1735, that wealth began to widen the family horizons. From modest merchant enterprises in Newport, Gibbs soon expanded his business to Connecticut and Massachusetts. Eventually worldwide trade was his concern.[2]

In October 1768, George Gibbs II married Mary Channing. The marriage soon resulted in a partnership between Gibbs and his wife's brother, Walter Channing. Under the name of Gibbs and Channing the brothers-in-law extended their economic activities.[3] By the time of the birth of the third George Gibbs, Newport, the firm's headquarters, was a busy trading town. It was the only accessible port in the region when strong winds blew from the northwest. In spite of these gusts, regular trade winds in winter, the harbor was a secure anchorage for vessels of any tonnage. Rhode Island's mild climate and proximity to the Gulf Stream also insured that Newport possessed an ice-free roadstead. The great ropewalks whose tarry odors perfumed the town, the seamen going up and down Mary Street bearing hempen cables for their ships, and the chimney sweeps moving among the clapboard houses clustered along the cobbled streets shouting 'sweep-ho!' gave the town a unique character.

The Gibbs and Channing fortune was derived from turtles and wines, both of which appealed to the appetites of New Englanders. To the shops on Thames Street the firm's ships brought turtles for soups and the vintage wines of Madeira and Cadiz. Despite the tribulations of the Revolutionary War, the Gibbs and Channing business waxed stronger, until by the 1790s it had nine sailing ships, three brigs, and the schooner *Federal* under its flag. The vessels regularly sailed to Batavia, the Isle of Bourbon, Havana, Surinam, Sweden, Russia, and Denmark.[4]

Such trading interests were a powerful force in the daily life of the Gibbs family. The excitement of foreign lands, the tales of the firm's captains such as the adventurer John Boit who as early as 1792 pioneered in the North Pacific sea otter trade, and the increasing profits all tended to develop awareness and sophistication in the Gibbs children. With the hope that his son would enter his firm's operations, in 1796 the elder Gibbs sent George Gibbs on a voyage half way around the world. The young man had seven months at sea on a company vessel before arriving in Macao and Canton to do business. From Canton on 11 November 1796, George wrote his father: 'Though the voyage is not likely to be of any considerable importance to me, you may depend on my utmost exertion in the management of the concerns entrusted to us, and I shall take care not to forfeit the character I derive from being, all with respect, your affectionate son.'[5]

In spite of his disclaimer the voyage was one of consequence; it helped Gibbs resolve to find pursuits other than commerce for his life's undertaking. The collapse of the market in Charleston, South Carolina, the destination of many of the goods he had secured in the Orient, was in 1797 further disillusionment for the young man.[6] Although financial speculation was not an excitement for him, travel was. Shortly after he received an M.A. degree from Brown University in 1800, Gibbs left for an extended tour of Europe. In the spring of 1801 he was in Paris; that summer he went to Russia to see the coronation of the Czar. During 1802 he resided at Berlin. Finally in 1803 Gibbs returned to Rhode Island with chests of minerals which he had collected during his excursions abroad.[7]

Col. George Gibbs's wanderlust and lack of interest in the family enterprises prompted, on 5 October 1803, a deathbed letter of instruction from his father:

It is time my Son, that you give up travelling, that you fix yourself to business & lead a regular life observing the strictest economy; for the person who lives beyond his income, will more than probable live to see the end of his property, without which, life indeed would be miserable. I have cancelled all demands in the company books against you, and left a portion equal with the other children. . . . Remember my Son, that as the dying request of a Parent, that you do in future regularly attend Church, reverence Religion and observe its holy & wise precepts, which alone can afford you peace of mind in the last hour.[8]

While the elder Gibbs's advice was well intentioned, his cancelling of his son's debts and liberal provision for him in his will were little inducement to draw the young man into the firm. Walter Channing and his widowed sister saw things realistically. In 1804 they began to liquidate vessels and inventories, to invest in less speculative but potentially profitable real estate, and to make the company manageable for a widow and an aging surviving partner.[9]

No doubt these decisions pleased Colonel Gibbs, for they meant that his mother would continue to have steady income and that he was free from any commitment that required his labor in Newport. More than symbolic of Mary Gibbs's security was her purchase in 1805 of the Harrison Gray Otis mansion constructed by the architect Charles Bulfinch on Mount Vernon Street near the State House in Boston.[10] She was secure financially and socially. The marriage of her nephew William Ellery Channing to her daughter, Ruth Gibbs, and their removal to her household in Boston, where Channing created a theological earthquake with his Unitarian preaching, brought the family into the mainstream of New England intellectual life.

American interest in geology was increasing during Gibbs's youth. As early as 1794 David Hosack imported from Europe a mineral collection that he exhibited in New York. Adam Seybert collected a cabinet that he brought to Philadelphia between 1795 and 1800. In New York, Samuel L. Mitchell, editor of the *Medical Repository*, first tried to organize interest in the subject when in 1799 he formed the short-lived American Mineralogical Society. Mitchell's cabinet and that started by Prof. Benjamin Waterhouse of Harvard University testified to the burgeoning interest in mineral specimens. That interest was furthered when in 1802 Benjamin D. Perkins returned from Europe with a cabinet and in 1803 when Archibald Bruce returned with his collection of minerals made during his European travels.[11]

Bruce, in particular, set a style for American scholars. He went to Europe in 1798, completed a medical degree at Edinburgh, and then in 1800 embarked on three years of wandering and studying with the leading geologists of the time. In London, Bruce visited Count de Bournon, the French exile who was cataloging the Greville mineral collection. In Paris he conferred with the Abbe Haüy. At Lausanne he studied with Heinrich Struve.[12]

Colonel Gibbs pursued a similar pattern of travel and study. While he apparently did not enroll in any institution, he studied extensively with some of the same geological luminaries that would later attract Bruce. Gibbs became well acquainted with the Abbe René Just Haüy and, in later years, was a dedicated user of the French savant's systems of nomenclature. Gibbs also studied in Lausanne with Struve. His travels took him on mineralogical expeditions to the Ardennes. There in 1805 he found a great mass of iron which he estimated at 3,400 pounds. In Paris he examined the collection of Gigot D'Orcy and in Switzerland met the renowned Russian geologist Count Grégoire Razamowsky.[13]

At the end of his second European sojourn in 1805, Gibbs engineered a great coup for American science made possible by his personal wealth. His father's death provided him with ample funds; the death of D'Orcy meant one major cabinet was for sale, and Gibbs's friendship with Razamowsky convinced the Russian to sell part of his collection. On Gibbs's return to the United States in 1805 he brought to Rhode Island the largest mineral cabinet then assembled in North America.

Heralded as 'Gibbs's grand Collection of Minerals,' the cabinet was described glowingly by the editor of the *Medical Repository* in 1808:

> This rich collection consists of the cabinets possessed by the late Mons. Gigot D'Orcy, of Paris, and the Count Grégoire de Razamowsky, a Russian nobleman, long resident in Switzerland. To which the present proprietor has added a number, either by himself on the spot, or purchased in different parts of Europe.
>
> The collection of Mr. D'Orcy is particularly rich in the productions of the French mines: Such as the phosphates, carbonates, and the mylydates of lead; the iron ores of Bangory, Framont, and Isle of Elba; the silver of St. Maria and d'Allemont; the mercury of Deuxponts; a great variety of marbles; calcedonies and agates, quartz, calcareous, and other spars from France and different parts of Europe.
>
> The collection of the Count Razamowsky consists chiefly of the minerals of the Russian empire. It is particularly rich in gold and copper ores, chromates of lead, the native iron of Pallas, Beryls, Jaspers, &c. The Russian specimens alone are about six thousand in number. The remainder are chiefly German and Swiss.

To these Mr. Gibbs has added all the newly discovered minerals, a complete collection of English, Swiss, and Italian specimens, including the ancient marbles, porphyries, &c. the muriates and carbonates of copper from Chili; the spinel and oriental rubies, of which this is the third complete collection existing. Also, a large geological collection. The whole consists of about twenty thousand specimens. . . .

In giving this account of a collection, so much wished for in the United States, it may be justly acknowledged, that it is principally by the assistance of the scavans of France, that it was rendered so complete; and that if it should prove useful to our country, the proprietor will share the pleasure with De L'Aumont, Daubuisson, Struve, and Bournon.[14]

For the young man from Newport the adventures in Europe had been of major importance. Not only had he made significant scientific friendships abroad, he had returned as a powerful force in American science. His homecoming in 1805 was hastened in part by the lament of his sister who had written to him in Paris that 'the responsibility on my Uncle is so great that it renders Mama very unhappy.' Family business thus caught up with the Colonel and brought him once again to Rhode Island.[15]

Others came to Newport as well, for as soon as Gibbs could unpack the cases containing his minerals and organize his collection, he was visited by eager mineralogists. He opened part of his cabinet in the summer of 1807 for study by friends and associates. Soon a young professor from Yale College, Benjamin Silliman, was eagerly trekking to Newport to study the collection. Silliman spent most of the summers of 1807 and 1808 working with the cabinet and exploring Rhode Island with the Colonel. The ties developing between the professor and the owner of the finest mineral collection in the country boded well for Yale's program in the sciences.[16] Yale's award to Gibbs in 1808 of an honorary Master of Arts degree helped to cement the bonds.[17]

The role which Gibbs so early assumed in American science was attested to in 1807 when Dr. Archibald Bruce, newly appointed professor of mineralogy in the State University of New York, wrote to Gibbs at the behest of Count Bournon:

It has been to me a source of regret to think that in this extensive and interesting tho unexplored country so little attention has been hitherto paid to Mineralogy. I trust however you will be the means of giving a spur to inquiry and that we shall have reason to acknowledge our obligations to you for the attention you have paid and the trouble you have taken to introduce among us a taste for this truly interesting and beautiful science.[18]

In his relationships with many Americans such as Bruce, Gibbs held the stature of master. Those who corresponded with him were his eager pupils. As the fame of his Newport cabinet spread, the letters and visitors increased. Some, such as Bruce, volunteered 'to communicate any information in my power respecting the Mineralogy of our vicinity and to send you such specimens as it affords.'[19] Others came in person to view the minerals, to borrow Gibbs's copies of the *Journal des Mines,* to see the latest works of Haüy, or to beg the loan of laboratory equipment.[20]

Where new directions beckoned, Gibbs frequently followed. Such was the case when in 1807 Silvain Godon, a Parisian mineralogist, emigrated to the United States and secured appointment to arrange the collections of the American Philosophical Society. Within a year of his arrival Godon published a notice in the *Medical Repository* about tourmalines. These semiprecious minerals had caught the interest of many because of their alleged electrical properties. When Godon suggested that in New Hampshire the 'mountains can easily furnish tourmalines enough for all the mineralogical collections in the world,' it was a challenge to any active collector to try that field.[21]

George Gibbs had special concerns that drew him into the wilds of America. His father had invested in mining properties, so Gibbs had inherited interests that called for management.[22] Further, the *Annals* of the American Academy and the work *American Geography* had both proclaimed that West River Mountain was volcanic. Suspecting that these statements were erroneous, but perhaps hopeful of finding tourmalines, Gibbs made an expedition to the White Mountains of New Hampshire during the summer of 1809.[23] The scope of his undertaking and the liberality with which he expended money to carry it out were attested to in 1816 when Jacob Bigelow, lecturer in materia medica and botany at Harvard University, described his own expedition in the same mountainous region. Of the zone of thickly entangled dwarf evergreens just below the summit on Mt. Washington Bigelow wrote:

> This zone of evergreens, has always constituted one of the most serious difficulties in the ascent of the White Hills. The passage through them is now much facilitated by a path cut by the direction of Col. Gibbs who ascended the mountain some years since.[24]

The expedition of 1809 enabled Gibbs to reject authoritatively volcanic activity in West River Mountain. He found no traces of recent eruption, located only granite and gneiss, found a small shaft on the mountain's summit where iron quarrying had once been undertaken, and put down the tales of a rumbling volcano as the work of local superstition.[25]

By 1810 Benjamin Silliman's interest in the Gibbs cabinet and his friendship with the Colonel were so great as to enable Silliman to persuade the wealthy mineralogist to deposit his collections in Yale College for use by the students in the scientific courses.[26] In May 1811 the negotiations for the transfer were underway. The question of proper storage, display, and controlled use were pressing issues for Silliman. Initially he contemplated cases to run the entire thirty-six feet of one wall of the mineralogical classroom. The bulk of the collection was impressive. The shipments from Newport to New Haven in November included fifty cartons and three barrels.[27]

Not only did Gibbs lend his collections, he became a patron of Yale's developing program of science instruction. In 1811, he began to offer an annual prize to a member of the Senior Division of the mineralogical class who won election by his peers. The prize consisted of 100 specimens taken from duplicates in his collection. One journal noted: 'The choice is founded upon superiority of attainments in mineralogical knowledge, and upon services rendered to the science by useful discoveries and observations.' In 1812 Silliman expanded the prize to include the Junior Division and accompanied it with free subscriptions to the *American Mineralogical Journal* and free admission to his courses in mineralogy.[28]

Gibbs's contributions to American science were, however, far more than that of generous patron of Silliman's programs of mineralogy and geology at Yale. His stature and role as participant and supporter of mineralogy appeared in his contributions to the *American Mineralogical Journal*. Archibald Bruce's zeal for a professional magazine to publish materials on American investigations became a reality in January 1810. Although the magazine was to last but a few years, its columns enabled American scientists to pursue their studies and compare their observations and discoveries.

The potential of such scientific undertakings was laid dramatically before the country on the evening of 14 December 1807. A meteor streaked across Long Island Sound and, to some Connecticut observers, seemed to explode overhead. Fragments showered to the earth to lodge in barnyards, gardens, and hillsides. Silliman hurried to the scene to gather specimens and to record eyewitness accounts of the phenomenal event. After analyzing the physical and chemical properties of the fragments early in 1808, he and James U. Kingsley wrote up the

observations and published them in 1810 in the *Memoirs* of the
Connecticut Academy of Science. The authors found the meteor
material granular and coarse. The particles were 'somewhat irregular,
like crystals of schorl,' noted Silliman.[29]

Such a meteor fall did not go unnoticed by Colonel Gibbs. He
purchased the largest meteor fragment, weighing nearly thirty-seven
pounds, from one of the keen-eyed farmers who had collected it.[30] In a
letter published in 1810 Gibbs did not vacillate about the properties of
the meteor. 'In examining some of the meteoric stones which fell at
Weston,' he wrote, 'I found imbedded in one of them a cubic crystal of
Pyrites about 2-3ds of an inch over, and at one angle of it another like
Crystal.' He boldly asserted: 'This discovery proves the existence of
crystallized bodies in the meteoric stones, which before had been only
conjectured by Mr. Gillet de l'Aumont of Paris, a distinguished French
mineralogist.' For Gibbs the presence of crystalline matter in a meteor
was of special significance because it brought into question the then
popular theory that meteors formed in the atmosphere.[31]

A second meteorite also attracted Gibbs's attention. In 1808 a
trader among the Pawnee Indians learned of a curious mass of iron
found by those people. His reports sent two rival parties rushing to
Louisiana in 1810 to recover the meteorite. The successful searchers
loaded the iron mass on a wagon and pulled it with a team of six horses
to the Mississippi where it was carried by boat to New Orleans. It too
was purchased by Gibbs for his cabinet. Immediately the question
arose whether the newly discovered substance was, as Gibbs phrased it,
a 'production of art or nature.'[32]

Silliman and Gibbs began an analysis of the mass and discovered
nickel and iron. The finding of nickel was, in Gibbs's view, authority
for natural origin. The investigators continued their work and placed
their iron extracts in nitric acid. 'You will easily conceive my surprise
in finding two of these pieces crystallized in the interior of octahedrons,
like the magnetic iron ore (*fer oxydule* of Haüy),' wrote Gibbs to Bruce.
He continued:

> They have the same characters as the rest of the mass in which they are
> imbedded, being only semi-hard, and easily cut with a knife, and some
> interstices appear between the lamina which mark the decroissemens, as is
> often observed in the crystals of the magnetic ore. The largest crystal was
> more than half an inch long.[33]

In his report on the Louisiana meteorite for the *American Miner-*
alogical Journal, Gibbs revealed the breadth of his mineralogical

studies. He compared his new specimen to the Siberian meteorite found by Pallas. That mass he had personally studied. He also made reference to the one described by DeCelis in South America, another by Chaladni of Magdeburg, and others found in Senegal, Hungary, and Thuringia. While he was even more convinced of the crystalline nature of meteorites, Gibbs was still uncertain about their formation. 'I should therefore be inclined to adopt the theory of celestial origin for some of those masses,' he noted, 'and that of the volcanic for others.' He was willing to leave the final statement on the subject to 'abler pens and more willing minds.'[34]

Many of Gibbs's interests were practical and utilitarian. Indeed among American men of science in the first two decades of the nineteenth century, Gibbs certainly deserved praise for seeking applications of advances in chemistry and mineralogy. Occasionally his views were merely practical and of interest only to colleagues. Such was his recommended change in nomenclature in delineating three distinct subspecies of native iron.[35] Other opinions related directly to the nation's economy and its growing industrial development.

Bruce's second number of the *American Mineralogical Journal* carried, perhaps at Gibbs's instigation, Albert Gallatin's 'Report of the Secretary of the Treasury on the State of American Manufacturing in 1810.' The account revealed that nearly 80 per cent of the bar iron used annually in the United States was of American manufacture and that the product was of inferior quality. In 1809 Gibbs had visited the iron smelter at Vergennes, Vermont and in January 1810, he examined the Franconia Iron Works in the Connecticut River Valley. The commercial potential of these enterprises probably attracted him and he noted that the venture at Franconia was capitalized at $100,000, had one furnace, four forges, and two workshops in operation. He examined the ores used by the smelter and wrote:

> The mineral is the magnetic iron ore (fer oligisle of Haüy). It is found compact, and fine grained. —The colour is a bluish grey, the powder nearly black; this ore is similar to the Swedish, and the same species which furnishes Europe and America with their best iron. In the same bed is found an abundance of crystallized and amorphous Red Garnet, Epidote of a light yellow colour, and Amphibole.[36]

As a field worker, Gibbs's breadth of experience and ability to ascertain the situation were impressive. More important, however, was his ability to assess the technological defects in the Franconia works. He found that the furnace was only twenty-six feet high; the ones he had observed in Europe were nearly twice the height. He knew that the less pure ores such as those in the Connecticut Valley needed more gradual heat. 'This is the effect of the high furnace,' he wrote, 'as it takes one-third more time for the ore to descend to the blast. It is then necessary to roast the ore, and the remnant of sulphur is disengaged more freely, and other foreign substances evaporated or scorified.' He further pointed out that a higher furnace meant a greater diameter with less heat loss and greater yield. He recommended that American production could be further improved with the building of furnaces with but one opening for drawing off the metal and scories.[37]

The Vergennes, Vermont operation was financed by Boston entrepreneurs. The company was tapping ores at Monckton and transporting them seven miles to the furnace. Here, too, Gibbs found faulty construction responsible for the poor quality of the product, though the ores were some of the finest he knew of in the United States. Not only was the furnace too short, it did not have straight sides as in Europe. He recommended reconstruction of the furnaces and inviting an expert from Europe to oversee the changes. 'The great fault of most of our manufactures,' he wrote, 'has been the employment of men without experience, or without the usage of the modern improvements. I know of none which have failed from any other cause.'[38]

The interest which Gibbs's travels and publications brought to the condition of bar iron manufacture was revealed when in March 1812 William Smith of Quebec submitted to the *American Mineralogical Journal* an article analyzing the iron works at Three Rivers in Canada. That he bothered to give the height of the furnace was evidence of his awareness of Gibbs's pronouncements on the subject.[39]

Gibbs's American travels were varied and extensive. On some of them he was accompanied by James Pierce, a wandering geologist who in later years was a frequent contributor to Silliman's *Journal*. Gibbs, however, found an even more interesting companion when in 1810 he married sixteen-year-old Laura Wolcott. The daughter of Oliver Wolcott, Secretary of the Treasury in the administrations of Washington and Adams, Laura had a sophistication fostered by long association with the country's leading citizens. At an early age she had served as her father's hostess. She accompanied her husband on several of his expeditions and took advantage of sojourns in the wilderness to discover new varieties of flowers or to sketch.[40]

Gibbs's social and professional ties were extensive. His mother's home in Boston drew him into the inner circle of Beacon Hill society. His long residence in Newport, his service as aide-de-camp to the state's governor, and the large scale of his father's business interests gave him many opportunities in Rhode Island. His own commercial interests drew him frequently to New York City. In 1809 he was nominated for membership in the socially select New York Historical Society and joined S. L. Mitchell, Archibald Bruce, David Hosack, and De Witt Clinton on its Natural History Committee. In later years he headed its Mineralogical Committee and contributed specimens to the collections which were eventually transferred to the cabinet of the New York Lyceum of Natural History.[41]

In 1811 Gibbs's stature in America was further recognized with his nomination and election to the American Philosophical Society. The following year he was named to the newly formed American Antiquarian Society and was elected one of the organization's seven vice-presidents. In 1813 he was elected to serve on the committee seeking information on the mounds and monuments of the Ohio Valley. In August 1813 he was elected to the American Academy of Arts and Sciences. The Academy of Natural Sciences of Philadelphia and the Linnaean Society of New England extended him membership in 1815.[42]

By 1813 Gibbs's interests and tastes were changing from science to more domestic concerns. In late 1813 he purchased a 140-acre estate at Hurlgate on Long Island. The farm faced the East River opposite Manhattan. An aspiring country squire, he named his property 'Sunswick Farms' and began early in 1814 major renovation of the eighteenth-century farmhouse, planting orchards, laying out gardens, and securing fine breeds of sheep and cattle. The extent of Gibbs's finances was shown by the $40,000 he paid for his new farm and the assets of $57,114 he had on account with his father-in-law Wolcott by the summer of 1814.[43]

The Colonel's fortunes had been spectacularly enlarged by one of his scientific associates. Robert Gilmore, Baltimore businessman, world traveler, and avid mineralogist, frequently purchased lottery tickets for Gibbs. The gamble on the Washington Monument Lottery was not productive, but his purchase for Gibbs of tickets in Baltimore's Vaccine Lottery yielded a windfall. On 23 November 1813, about the time Gibbs was negotiating for the Long Island estate, Gilmore wrote that to the great dismay of the citizens of Maryland, Gibbs had won $30,000 in the lottery. He added: 'If your mineralogical excursions turn out so well, you will really have found the Philosophers Stone, and made gold from our base hills. . . .'[44]

At his new headquarters on Long Island, Gibbs set up a laboratory, unpacked his books and instruments, and maintained a small cabinet of select minerals. As he had in past years greeted scientific associates and helped supply struggling professors with specimens, crucibles, and publications, so he continued at Sunswick. John Torrey, for example, wrote to Amos Eaton in June 1819:

> I am now thick with Gibbs—he is a princely fellow. He lives 7 or 8 miles from here (on Long Island) & has a fine laboratory, well furnished. I shall go there to analyze my Datholite & his Brucite (Fluate of Magnesia & Silex). He gives me many minerals.[45]

Occasionally Gibbs's largess was of a very practical nature. Constantine Rafinesque, naturalist and writer, begged Gibbs in May 1817 to help him raise additional bond. 'If I am not too presuming,' he petitioned, 'could I crave you to confer on me a further obligation by standing bail again, as I have no body to whom to apply more properly just now.'[46]

One of Gibbs's most frequent correspondents was Prof. Parker Cleaveland of Bowdoin College in Brunswick, Maine. Their relationship was fostered by exchange of minerals and by Cleaveland's ardent strivings to develop a competency in mineralogy. On one occasion, having obtained permission to blast rocks for emeralds, the exultant professor proclaimed: 'If successful, je pouvrai partager avec vous le fruit.'[47] Cleaveland suffered from his impecunious post and his distance from the fellowship of active mineralogists. He frequently wrote to Silliman and implored the Yale professor to rally support for a geological society. In the fall of 1813 Cleaveland wrote to Gibbs: 'After consulting with Prof. Silliman I have begun the preparation of an elementary work on Mineralogy & Geol[ogy] to be comprised in a single volume. The need of such a work is very sensibly felt by instructors, and it may probably tend to a more general diffusion of mineralogical knowledge, as all the valuable systems, we now have, are contained in from 2 to 5 volumes.'[48]

Silliman steadfastly advised Cleaveland that he must, if he were to persist in writing the text, travel to New Haven to study the Gibbs cabinet. 'I have long most ardently desired to see that Cabinet,' he lamented to Gibbs, 'and nothing but the great length of the Journey, and my own poverty have hitherto prevented.'[49] Through 1814 and 1815 Cleaveland labored on his volume and frequently importuned Gibbs and Silliman for specific locations of mineral deposits to aid the field worker. 'It is not for myself,' he wrote, 'it is for the convenience of pupils and for the progress of the science, that I plead.'[50]

Although Gibbs corresponded freely and warmly with Cleaveland, Torrey, Eaton, Maclure, and Gilmore, his most enduring allegiance was to his friend Benjamin Silliman. Silliman continued to find significant specimens and convinced Gibbs to purchase them for the collections at Yale. He borrowed copies of Haüy, Brochant, Cuvier, Bakewell, and the *Journal des Mines*.[51] On one occasion he requested 'two dozen of the black lead pots or crucibles in the sizes the largest about No. 8 or 9—viz. to contain 3 pints or a quart & so down to the smallest size.'[52] He shared with Gibbs his teaching plans and the development of new courses. In February 1816, for example, Silliman wrote to his friend:

> I am thinking of attempting to render the course of mineralogical Instruction more complete by giving a course of about 20 lectures on the analysis of minerals; if given they will come immediately at the conclusion of the chemical course & of the private mineralogical lectures. Do you know of any manual better than Accum's?[53]

Their mutual interests led to the establishment of the *American Journal of Science* under Silliman's editorial control in 1818. Gibbs's strongly applied scientific approach was evident in the journal's prefatory 'Plan of the Work.' The new publication was to cover all the physical sciences 'with their application to the Arts, and to every useful purpose.' The full intent was clearly enunciated:

> While Science will be cherished *for its own sake*, and with due respect for its own *inherent* dignity; it will also be employed as the *handmaid to the Arts*. Its numerous applications to Agriculture, the earliest and most important of them; to Manufactures, both mechanical and chemical; and to our Domestic Economy, will be carefully sought out, and faithfully made.[54]

By February 1818, Silliman had a prospectus for the journal ready to distribute to interested subscribers. Gibbs received a number of them to distribute in Boston and Cambridge. Silliman urged him to get them to the Athenaeum, the Exchange Coffee House, and to the principal booksellers. The proposal for the journal gained good response. By May, Silliman reported 412 subscribers and thought that he could probably raise it to 500.[55]

Gibbs wrote an article on practical application of science for the first number. He based it on careful observations made during improvements on his estate in the fall of 1817. Having a worker blasting rocks, Gibbs decided to test a newly suggested procedure. Employing one part quicklime to two parts of gunpowder, he found 'the same charge to answer equally well with a like quantity of gunpowder.' Several experiments with the procedure revealed to him, however, that the mixing of ingredients had to be done on the day of blasting. He observed that the quicklime absorbed moisture and aided immediate detonation. If the mixture stood for several hours, however, Gibbs noted that the lime attacked the water crystallization of the saltpeter and diminished the power of the charge. He reported that the heat of a cannon probably worked similarly as a desiccating agent through volatilizing moisture in the gunpowder.[56]

More speculative and revealing of his knowledge of trends in scientific investigation was Gibbs's article for Silliman 'On the Connexion Between Magnetism and Light.' He explained that a friend in New Jersey had discovered that his mine sometimes yielded iron ores without magnetism when quarried a hundred feet beneath the surface. Gibbs knew that the renowned Abraham Werner of the School of Mines at Freiberg in Saxony had reported a similar discovery. Suspecting that an atmospheric or cosmic factor caused polarity, Gibbs stated: 'The late discovery of the magnetic influence of the violet rays of light, by Morechini, a notice of which has since reached us in the journals, connected with the above fact, leads me to believe that light is the great source of magnetism.' To support his proposal, Gibbs discussed Herschel's discovery of the rays invisible to human sight and noted their property of refraction. Suspecting great light refraction in the polar regions and linking this to his theory that light induced magnetism, Gibbs was able to suggest that this was the probable cause of the magnetic poles in those areas. To make his proposition even more provocative, he concluded that polar ice and snow probably emitted magnetic rays that with electricity 'may, perhaps, give us the aurora borealis.'[57]

Silliman published the speculative paper and later printed Gibbs's note on an experiment that he had performed using his magnet. By exposing the magnet to light, Gibbs wrote, he had found that it gained twelve ounces of power with forty minutes of exposure. Neither of Gibbs's magnetism articles of 1818 led to scientific breakthroughs. Were they taken seriously, they either produced some lively experimentation or some agonizing frustration.[58]

The rebirth in America of a journal which focused on the physical sciences and especially mineralogy and geology was but one sign of the discipline's maturation. By 1818 Dr. J. W. Webster returned from two years of study in Europe, where he had accumulated a sizable cabinet, to commence teaching mineralogy at Harvard. Gibbs aided Webster in establishing and ordering the collections at Cambridge.[59] These interests led in 1819 to serious discussions for developing a professional organization. Silliman wrote to Gibbs in February: 'It strikes me that it will be better to have the society mineralogical & geological but I have not thought deeply on that point.' By March Gibbs's plans for the organization had been circulated. Silliman told him: 'I like all your suggestions as to the G[eological] Soc[iety]. Mr. Bruce has written me & is much pleased. Cleaveland also expresses himself gratified.' For Silliman the choice of a president was between Gibbs or William Maclure. Should Maclure win, he noted to Gibbs, 'You must be first V.P. which will make you really the acting P[resident].' Silliman's supposition that Maclure would probably decline because of his frequent visits abroad did not materialize. When the American Geological Society formed in the rooms of Yale College on 6 September 1819, Maclure became President, Gibbs First Vice-President, Silliman Second Vice-President, and Cleaveland Third Vice-President. Members included Constantine Rafinesque, Robert Hare, Robert Gilmore, and Silvain Godon—that loose circle of friends that for more than a decade had sparked the study of geology in the United States.[60]

The respect that Gibbs had earned among those colleagues was attested to in 1820 when Amos Eaton published the second edition of his *Index to the Geology of the Northern States,* dedicated to George Gibbs. Eaton heralded Silliman's instruction and the Gibbs cabinet as essential to the realization of the volume.[61] To John Torrey in February 1820 Eaton wrote: 'Gibbs will always be remembered in this country as the father of *correct* American geology. There were some pretty good mineralogists before he began; but his cabinet first set us all off to work, hunting up our own minerals. Besides his own exertions, you know, are unequalled.'[62]

Friend, patron, and correspondent, George Gibbs inspired many of America's early men of science. Through the 1820s he continued to review articles for Silliman before they were published in the *American Journal of Science.*[63] He donated specimens, maps, books, minerals, and equipment, and he received additional honors. The memberships included the Société Française de Statistique Universelle of Paris and the Agricultural Society of Vienna.[64]

As the years passed Gibbs's personal affairs weighed increasingly upon him. He and Laura had seven children. Their needs and education required his time and money. His decision in 1824 to send his eldest son, George, to the experimental Round Hill School in the Connecticut Valley evidenced his interest in progressive education. His attempt to win appointment from President Monroe as Minister to Mexico was unrealized.[65] Gibbs found himself, instead, compelled in 1820 to mortgage his estate for $12,000. Unable to pay off this amount to his creditor by 1824, he was ready to dispose of his mineral collection.[66] Thus it was that Silliman rallied Yale's alumni and friends to secure $20,000 to pay Gibbs for the cabinet that had trained students for a decade and a half. The purchase was completed in May 1824.[67] The death of Gibbs's mother, Mary Channing Gibbs, on 26 December that same year solved the Colonel's financial concerns.[68]

Generous giving, gambling, and a taste for luxurious living were factors in the life of Col. George Gibbs. His patronage of the arts included several commissions to his lifelong friend Gilbert Stuart. Gibbs owned portraits of himself and his wife by Stuart and, at one time, also possessed the second portrait that the artist had done from life of George Washington. Eventually when Gibbs disposed of that art work, he had Stuart paint for him the set of five presidential portraits, likenesses of Washington, Adams, Jefferson, Madison, and Monroe.[69]

On 5 August 1834 Gibbs died at Sunswick Farms, aged fifty-seven years.[70] He was survived by his wife and young family. Benjamin Silliman eulogized him in the *American Journal of Science* by noting: 'His talents were decidedly of a superior order; his knowledge was extensive and various; his style of writing was simple, concise, and comprehensive, and his original observations were judicious and exact.'[71] His life had been pleasant. He had lived with fortune and friendship. Had he possessed less of either, perhaps George Gibbs might have embraced the world of science with even greater passion and striven more diligently to master the secrets of nature. The lure of mineralogy and geology had, however, considerably deepened his life, and his wisdom and generosity enabled others to walk through the doors that he opened.

NOTES

[1]Obituary of Col. George Gibbs, *Am. J. Sci.*, 1834, 25, 215.

[2]Gibbs, *Gibbs Family*.

[3]Channing, *Early Recollections of Newport*, pp. 133–134.

[4]*Ibid.*, pp. 136–137.

[5]George Gibbs, Jr. to George Gibbs, 11 November 1796, Gibbs Manuscripts, Madison.

[6] Rogers, Barker & Lord to Gibbs, 11 September 1797, Gibbs Manuscripts, Madison.

[7] George Barclay to Gibbs, 17 March 1801; J. G. Proud to Gibbs, 21 September 1801; Gibbs to Appleton, 3 January 1802; William Powell to Gibbs, 24 August 1803, Gibbs Manuscripts, Madison.

[8] George Gibbs, Jr. to George Gibbs, 5 October 1803, Gibbs Manuscripts, Madison.

[9] Gibbs, *Gibbs Family*, pp. 15–16.

[10] Susan Parsons and Wendell D. Garrett, 'The Second Harrison Gray Otis House, Boston,' *Antiques*, 1967, *92*, 536–541.

[11] Review of P. Cleaveland's *Treatise on Mineralogy and Geology* in *Am. J. Sci.*, 1818, *1*, 37; 'Elegant and Instructive Collections of Minerals,' *Med. Repos., Philad.*, 1805, *2*, 433–434.

[12] Bruce to Gibbs, 10 July 1807, Gibbs Manuscripts, Newport; Obituary of Archibald Bruce, *Am. J. Sci.*, 1818, *1*, 301; *Am. mineral. J.*, John Greene's introduction to reprint vol. 1 (New York and London: Hafner Reprints, 1968), pp. vii–viii.

[13] Haüy to [?], 8 September 1807; Bruce to Gibbs, 10 July 1807, Gibbs Manuscripts, Newport; George Gibbs, 'Largest Mass of European Meteoric Iron,' *Edinb. phil. J.*, 1825, *13*, 186.

[14] 'Gibbs' Grand Collection of Minerals.' *Med. Repos., Philad.*, 1808, 2d Hexade, *5*, 213–214.

[15] Helen Eliza Gibbs to Gibbs, 22 June 1805, Wolcott-Gibbs Manuscripts, Eugene.

[16] Benjamin Silliman, 'Anthracite Coal of Rhode-Island,' *Am. J. Sci.*, 1826, *11*, 79.

[17] *Biographical Dictionary of America*, s. v. 'Gibbs, George.'

[18] Bruce to Gibbs, 10 July 1807, Gibbs Manuscripts, Newport.

[19] *Ibid.*

[20] *Ibid.*, 14 July and 2 August 1809; Silliman to Gibbs, 19 February 1808, Gibbs Manuscripts, Newport.

[21] 'American Tourmaline,' *Med. Repos., Philad.*, 1808, 2d Hexade, *5*, 307. In 1818 Gibbs published 'On the Tourmalines and other Minerals found at Chesterfield and Goshen, Massachusetts,' *Am. J. Sci.*, 1818, *1*, 346–351.

[22] Jonathan Allen, 'On the Question, whether there are any traces of a Volcano in the West River Mountain,' *Am. J. Sci.*, 1821, *3*, 73–74.

[23] George Gibbs, 'Mineralogical notice respecting the West River Mountain, Connecticut River,' *Am. mineral. J.*, 1810, *1*, 19.

[24] Jacob Bigelow, 'Some Account of the White Mountains of New Hampshire,' *New Eng. J. Med. Surg.*, 1816, *5*, 327.

[25] Gibbs, (n. 23), pp. 19–20.

[26] 'Cabinet of Minerals, at Yale College,' *Am. mineral. J.*, 1810, *1*, 126.

[27] Silliman to Gibbs, 10 May and 27 November 1811, Gibbs Manuscripts, Newport; Gibbs to Silliman, 12 March 1811, Gibbs Manuscripts, Madison.

[28] 'Mineralogical Premiums,' *Am. mineral. J.*, 1810, *1*, 269–270; Gibbs to Silliman, May 1811, Gibbs Manuscripts, Madison.

[29] 'An Account of the Meteor which burst over Weston in Connecticut, 14 December,

1807, and of the falling stones on that occasion,' *Mem. Conn. Acad. Arts Sci.*, 1810, *1*, 158.

[30] Silliman to Gibbs, 19 February 1808, Gibbs Manuscripts, Newport.

[31] 'Extract of a letter from Col. Gibbs, to the Editor,' *Am. mineral. J.*, 1810, *1*, 190.

[32] C. H., 'Notice of the Malleable Iron of Louisiana,' *Am. J. Sci.*, 1821, *8*, 219–221.

[33] George Gibbs, 'Observations on the Mass of Iron from Louisiana,' *Am. mineral. J.*, 1810, *1*, 218–219.

[34] *Ibid.*, pp. 219–221.

[35] 'Proposed Classification of some of the Ores of Iron,' *Am. mineral. J.*, 1810, *1*, 268.

[36] George Gibbs, 'Observations on the Franconia Iron Works,' *Am. mineral. J.*, 1810, *1*, 80–83.

[37] *Ibid.*, pp. 6–7.

[38] George Gibbs, 'On the Iron Works at Vergennes, Vermont,' *Am. mineral. J.*, 1810, *1*, 80–83.

[39] William Smith, 'Observations on the Saint Maurice iron works,' *Am. mineral. J.*, 1810, *1*, 198–199.

[40] *New Engl. hist. geneal. Reg.*, 1871, *25*, 309; Laura Gibbs to [?], 11 April 1811, Gibbs Manuscripts, Madison.

[41] *Coll. N.Y. hist. Soc.*, 1841, *2d ser. 1*, 465; Wilson, ed., *New-York*, III, 201.

[42] J. Vaughan to Gibbs, 4 February 1811, Gibbs Manuscripts, Madison; American Antiquarian Society, *Proceedings, 1812–1849*, p. 7; Josiah Quincy to Gibbs, 18 August 1813; Reuben Haines to Gibbs, 31 January 1815; Jacob Bigelow to Gibbs, 27 January 1815, Gibbs Manuscripts, Newport.

[43] Oliver Wolcott to Gibbs, 15 January and 28 January 1814, Wolcott-Gibbs Manuscripts, Eugene; George Gibbs, 'Accounts with Oliver Wolcott,' Gibbs Manuscripts, Newport.

[44] Robert Gilmore to Gibbs, 17 September 1812, 14 February and 23 November 1813, Gibbs Manuscripts, Newport.

[45] John Torrey to Amos Eaton, 16 June 1819, quoted in McAllister, *Eaton*, p. 264.

[46] Rafinesque to Gibbs, 14 May 1817, Gibbs Manuscripts, Newport.

[47] Cleaveland to Gibbs, 17 March 1810, Gibbs Manuscripts, Newport.

[48] *Ibid.*, 18 October 1813.

[49] *Ibid.*, 23 December 1813.

[50] *Ibid.*, 21 February 1816.

[51] Silliman to Gibbs, 27 April 1812, 3 May 1813, 12 January and 19 February 1816, Gibbs Manuscripts, Newport.

[52] *Ibid.*, 8 December 1814.

[53] *Ibid.*, 19 February 1816.

[54] 'Plan of the Work,' *Am. J. Sci.*, 1818, *1*, v–vi.

[55] Silliman to Gibbs, 26 February and 10 May 1818, Gibbs Manuscripts, Newport.

[56] George Gibbs, 'On a Method of Augmenting the Force of Gunpowder,' *Am. J. Sci.*, 1818, *1*, 87–88.

[57] George Gibbs, 'On the Connexion between Magnetism and Light,' *Am. J. Sci.*, 1818, *1*, 89-90.

[58] George Gibbs, 'Extract of a Letter,' *Am. J. Sci.*, 1818, *1*, 207.

[59] J. T. Kirkland to Gibbs, 19 January 1820, Gibbs Manuscripts, Newport; 'An Address to the People of the Western Country,' *Am. J. Sci.*, 1818, *1*, 204-206; 'Introductory Remarks' to a letter to the editor by William Maclure, *Am. J. Sci.*, 1818, *1*, 210.

[60] Silliman to Gibbs, 6 February and 17 March 1819, Gibbs Manuscripts, Newport; Merrill, *American Geology*, pp. 61-62.

[61] Eaton, *Geology of the Northern States*, p. iii.

[62] Eaton to Torrey, 27 February 1820, quoted in McAllister, *Eaton*, p. 264.

[63] 'Remarks,' *Am. J. Sci.*, 1822, *4*, 38; Editor's footnote, *Am. J. Sci.*, 1822, *4*, 253.

[64] Cesar Moreau to Gibbs, 10 April 1830; anonymous letter to Gibbs, 4 October 1824, Gibbs Manuscripts, Newport.

[65] Beckham, 'Gibbs,' pp. 14, 19-20.

[66] George Gibbs, 'Indenture of 10 March, 1820,' 'Indenture of 27 Nov. 1823,' Gibbs Manuscripts, Madison.

[67] E. Goodrich to Gibbs, 24 May 1824, Gibbs Manuscripts, Madison.

[68] Gibbs, *Gibbs Family*, p. 65.

[69] *Ibid.*, pp. 145-148; Park, *Stuart*, I, 348-349.

[70] George Gibbs, 'Surrogate Records,' 13 August 1833.

[71] Obituary of Col. George Gibbs, *Am. J. Sci.*, 1834, *25*, 214-215.

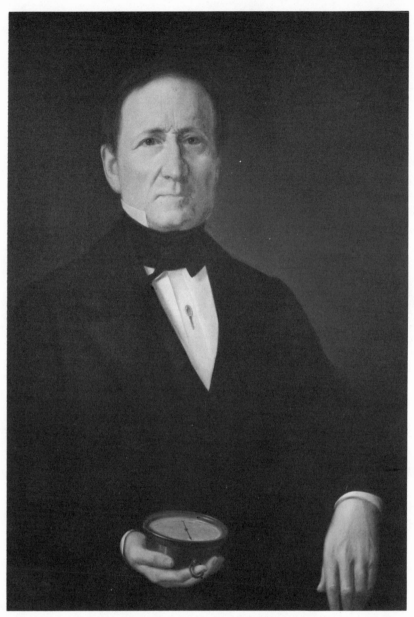

Edward Hitchcock, artist unknown.

Edward Hitchcock

GLORIA ROBINSON

THROUGH THE INFLUENCE of his students, the impress of
Benjamin Silliman's interests and endeavors on the development
of American science extended far beyond his own contributions. Across
a handwritten page of Silliman's 'Reminiscences' on which he
summed up the 'Results in Life' of his regular assistants who 'Became
Professors of Science' is this entry: 'Edward Hitchcock Amherst
College Prof^r Pres^t and Prof^r again.'[1]

Silliman wrote, 'His starting point was with us and we may regard
him as a pupil of our scientific departments.'[2] As a young theological
student Hitchcock heard Silliman's lectures, and later he was an
assistant in the chemistry laboratory. Their correspondence and friendship was lifelong.

Silliman first encouraged Hitchcock's interest in geology and
mineralogy, and Hitchcock contributed to Silliman's *Journal* from its
inception. Letters traveled back and forth between Amherst and New
Haven while Hitchcock, as a young minister, studied the Connecticut
River Valley, became professor of science, headed the geological survey
of the state of Massachusetts, investigated the mysterious footprints
in the new red sandstone of the Connecticut Valley, and became president of Amherst College, later to return entirely to teaching and his
research.

To both Silliman and Hitchcock, geology provided boundless
illustration of design and divine beneficence, transcending whatever
apparent difficulties might lie in the account in *Genesis*, and for both
men science, especially geology, was inseparable from religion and a
moral view of life.

The Amherst College library kindly permitted extensive use of the Special Collections, especially of the Hitchcock-Silliman correspondence; and I should like to thank
J. Richard Phillips and Diana Brown for their aid in these researches. All quotations
from the President Edward Hitchcock Papers are made with the permission of the
Trustees of Amherst College, as is the reproduction of the portrait of Edward Hitchcock
for which Lewis A. Shepard kindly arranged—this 'official' portrait is in the Johnson
Chapel at Amherst College. I should like to express my appreciation to the libraries of
Yale University for the opportunity to examine a range of manuscript material, and
permission to publish therefrom, and to thank Judith Schiff for help and advice in the
use of the Silliman Family Papers in the Manuscripts and Archives, Yale University
Library.

Silliman recalled his first acquaintance with young Hitchcock, who had sent him a box of minerals for identification from Deerfield, Massachusetts where he was principal of the academy.

> More than forty years ago, I believe in the year 1817, I received a box of minerals from a person then unknown to me, who signed his name Edward Hitchcock teacher of the Academy of Deerfield Mass. He stated that he had collected these minerals from the rocks and mountains in that vicinity and as he stated moreover that they were unknown to him, he desired me to name them and return them to him with the labels. I promptly complied with the request and as the accompanying letter of M[r] Hitchcock was written with modest good sense and indicated a love of knowledge I invited him to send me another box, and I promised him to return it with the information he desired. It came and was attended to accordingly.
>
> The minerals were chiefly of the zeolite family—chabasic analcime mezotype, & agatized quartz &c being the usual companions of trap rocks such as are numerous in that region. I then invited M[r] Hitchcock to visit me in New Haven. The invitation was accepted and for a series of years, he was often here, and attended all the courses of lectures, with more or less of regularity. He discovered an amiable character and an ardent mind, animated by the love of knowledge, & he engaged with great industry in the study of chemistry mineralogy and geology.[3]

But the extent of Silliman's kindness and support is more fully revealed in the letters that passed between Silliman and his scientific correspondent in Deerfield. From New Haven on 24 August 1817, Silliman wrote, 'Dear Sir, You will find I believe most of your questions answered in the memoranda in the box,' and told Hitchcock about the garnets and copper. Encouragingly, 'I am happy you are busying yourself with mineralogical and geological observations.' He was sending Hitchcock a specimen of his own, one of marble, and asked for certain specimens.[4] The next week a reply from Hitchcock thanked Silliman for adding to the box of minerals from his own collection. 'I received the box of minerals I requested you to name and feel very grateful to you for bestowing so much labor upon them and also for the valuable and unexpected addition you made to them from your own cabinet.'

He told Silliman of the geological map he was making of the Connecticut River Valley, and that he was sending mineralogical specimens, suggesting that Silliman keep some 'and only send back such as you please.'[5]

Silliman was interested in seeing Hitchcock's geological map.[6]

Then in confidence a few weeks later, Silliman wrote that he was
thinking of publishing a scientific journal and would be pleased to
include Hitchcock's work in the first issue.[7] According to Silliman's
record:

> The Journal of Science was instituted the next year 1818 and Mr Hitchcock
> appeared in the first volume. His communications have been numerous
> and important. I have found between fifty and sixty titles of his papers in
> the tables of contents and in the Index. Not a few of these are elaborate and
> indicate much care and skill.[8]

Silliman had recognized the unusual talent and perseverance that
had already made Hitchcock, in his modest way, a leader in his native
town of Deerfield. Born on 24 May 1793, Hitchcock was the son of
Mercy Hoyt Hitchcock and Justin Hitchcock, respected as a deacon of
the church at Deerfield, a veteran of the Revolutionary War, a farmer
and hatter. His parents were sensitive to Edward Hitchcock's needs but
could do little in their poverty for the education of their three sons.[9] By
day Edward worked on a farm his brother rented, but 'I had acquired a
strong relish for scientific pursuits and I seized upon every moment I
could secure—especially rainy days and evenings—for those studies.'[10]
Major-General Hoyt, an uncle, helped him in his study of astronomy
and natural philosophy, and Hitchcock used the instruments of the
academy to make extensive calculations on the comet of 1811.[11] Later,
over several years, Hitchcock achieved a minor renown as he repeatedly
unearthed errors in Edmund M. Blunt's *Nautical Almanac* through
careful calculations of his own—errors which eventually Blunt
grudgingly acknowledged. Nevertheless Blunt never made good on the
Almanac's repeated promise that 'ten dollars will be paid on the
discovery of an error in the figures.'[12]

Hitchcock participated in debating and in philosophical discussion with a group of friends, but his academic hopes were to receive
sharp disappointment. 'I aimed to fit myself to pass through Harvard
University,' he recalled in his *Reminiscences* years afterward, 'but
Providence first struck down my ability to study. . . .'[13] An attack of
mumps damaged his eyes and '. . . compelled me to suspend nearly all
study and to change the whole course of my life, abandoning a college
course as impracticable, and for a time nearly all hope of pursuing
science or literature as a profession.'[14]

In 1816 Hitchcock became principal of the Deerfield Academy, and
during his three years there began studying for the ministry. At first
because of his health, he became interested in natural history, influ-

enced by the lectures of Amos Eaton at Amherst: 'I always regarded him as the chief agent of introducing a taste for these subjects into the Connecticut Valley.'[15]

During their early correspondence Hitchcock's letters to Silliman tell of collecting minerals and of botanical excursions, and mention visits to New Haven:

> I return you my acknowledgements for your polite invitation to visit N. Haven again. It would be very gratifying to me to be there this summer and hear your lectures on Geology: But I am compelled to follow the dictates of necessity not my own inclination. But wherever I am be assured Sir, that your kindness and assistance to me will not soon be effaced from the mind of your humble servant.[16]

Then, undoubtedly through Silliman's efforts on Hitchcock's behalf, Yale granted Hitchcock an honorary M.A. On 28 September 1818, Hitchcock wrote of his surprise and appreciation:

> The unexpected conferring of a degree upon me by your college awakens within me the liveliest feelings of gratitude and I have much reason for supposing that you, Sir, have not been inactive in my favour. Having been completely frustrated in every effort to pass regularly through a college by weakness of sight and of constitution I had relinquished the idea of ever acquiring the honors of any, much less one so eminent as Yale. I fear that I shall never be able to make any adequate return for this favour; but I hope at least that a thankful heart will not fail me.[17]

Hitchcock left Deerfield Academy in 1818 to prepare for the ministry. He hoped to study at New Haven under Professor Fitch and to hear Silliman's geology lectures as well.[18] Silliman welcomed this arrangement. 'I did not know you had changed your pursuits. I am pleased to know that you will prosecute them here.—The lectures of every description will be perfectly acceptable to you.'[19]

While in New Haven, Hitchcock experienced a change in his religious views and found that the orthodox creed was not as intolerant as he had supposed.[20] Through Silliman's introduction to the new geology, Hitchcock was faced, like others in his time, with the need to reconcile the facts of geology with the biblical accounts. His discussions with Silliman were continued in their letters, as Silliman wrote: 'I think you get off well between Moses and the Divines. . . . I have become still more convinced of the truth of the new views and am satisfied that they will ultimately become general among men who are at once acquainted with geology and disposed to reverence the scriptures.'[21]

Both men saw the goodness of God in all of nature. Years before, Silliman, when changing professions and giving up the law for his appointment in science, had felt this to be a strong reason for his choice.

> On the other hand—the study of nature appeared very attractive. In her works there is no falsehood, although there are mysteries, to unveil which is a very interesting achievement. Everything in nature is straitforward and consistent; there are no polluting influences; all the associations with these pursuits are elevated and virtuous and point toward the infinite creator.[22]

Silliman had pointed out the connections between the aims of science and divine design in his introduction to the first volume of the *Journal.* 'In a word, the whole circle of physical science is directly applicable to human wants, and constantly holds out a light to the practical arts; it thus polishes and benefits society, and every where demonstrates both supreme intelligence, and harmony and beneficence of design in THE CREATOR.'[23]

Hitchcock, drawn to religion and to the study of nature, found them inseparable. He entered the pastorate in Conway, Massachusetts, near Deerfield, in June 1821[24] and meanwhile continued his local explorations, collecting fossil fish impressions in nearby Sunderland and sending them to Silliman for further advice and identification.[25] Eventually he became concerned that his interest in natural history might be affecting his religious sensibilities and the performance of his duties as a minister, 'As I write this Sabbath evening I take the liberty to propose to you a case of conscience. . . .'

But need his pursuits in geology and botany really interfere if they were carried on in a religious context? Hitchcock had struggled with this problem of conscience for which he sought Silliman's advice.

> So much so indeed sometimes as to make me fearful I was not in the way of duty and to suspect that I might be worshipping idols—and if these pursuits be the right eye that must be plucked out let them not be spared however painful the effort—Now the thought has occurred to me that you might have had the same trials to go through and therefore might be able to counsel me. Pray tell me if you can the remedy in such a case—Must these pursuits be altogether abandoned? or is there such a thing as pursuing them with a supreme reference to the glory of God? Or does the difficulty lie in attending to them too eagerly? I put these enquiries to you because a mere theologist it seems to me could not answer them satisfactorily—There is however this difference between your case & mine—you attend to these subjects professionally—I only relaxationally.[26]

Hitchcock had meantime been continuing his correspondence on science with Silliman, and Silliman, as he forwarded books and journals, was keeping Hitchcock well informed on current questions in geology in America and abroad. Hitchcock, however, on receiving German journals from Silliman, could but thank him for his 'kind intentions' and ask rather for English or perhaps French communications. 'I am wholly ignorant of that language & know of nobody in this region who is acquainted with it.'[27]

But Hitchcock was to take up the problem of reconciling religion and geology more directly, when in 1823 he gave a sermon, entitled 'Utility of Natural History,' before the newly founded Berkshire Medical Institution at Pittsfield, Massachusetts.[28] He expected repercussions but, as he wrote to Silliman whose arguments he had cited, 'Certainly if I am condemned they cannot deny I have good company.'[29] Accompanying some books he was returning to Silliman, Hitchcock's letter gave an account of this recent discourse.

> I lately preached a sermon before the Pittsfield Med. Institution in which I have come out with the new views in regard to the first chapter in Genesis. It is now in the press & I hope you will pardon me for referring to your Lectures as an instance of the defense of such views in this country. My statements must be propped up by some good authorities or they will be disregarded since our divines generally do not as you have remarked understand even the elements of the subject.[30]

In this sermon, Hitchcock proceeded from a discussion of the role of natural history and its 'utility . . . in demonstrating the existence of God,' to some of the views of geology, actually no longer novel, as he pointed out. These held that the fossil remains embedded in rock had required too long for their deposition to have been laid down in the biblical Flood; and that the formation of the secondary strata with their successive and characteristic assemblages of organized remains had taken place over a period far exceeding six days of creation as we measure them.

> The truth of this statement in regard to the remains of animals in secondary strata is unquestionable, and no geologist can suppose that immense mountains of rock could have been deposited, without a miracle, in six literal days. It would be a want of candour not to acknowledge that hundreds, not to say thousands, of years, were requisite to effect this stupendous work. To reconcile the facts then with the Mosaic account is the problem the Christian geologist has to resolve.[31]

There were alternative hypotheses—one proposed that a long

intermediate period had intervened between the first creation and the advent of man, which was the event far more crucial to revelation.

> The grand object of revelation is to give us the history of man from his first creation. And concerning the time in which he was formed there exists very little diversity of opinion—geologists of every name, infidel and Christian, generally agreeing, that the voice of nature unites with the history of all nations in testifying to the truth of the Scriptures that man has existed on the globe not more than five or six thousand years. . . . The question then whether the earth existed for a time previous to the creation of man becomes a speculative enquiry of little practical importance. . . . For it can never be shown that Moses fixes the exact time of the original creation of the globe, although he does that of the human race.[32]

Hitchcock could quote well-founded opinion that such views did not oppose the Mosaic account of the creation, since they acknowledged the Creator and sought only to explain 'secondary instruments,' and he cited Silliman's authority as well.

> Among those gentlemen in this country, who have publicly maintained sentiments similar to those given above, I trust I shall be pardoned in naming Professor Silliman; who, in his able and eloquent lectures on geology, has been for several years in the habit of illustrating and defending such views of this subject, with all that clearness and force which experience and accurate knowledge enable him to do: and it gives me pleasure to add, with all that zeal too, with which an ardent attachment to revealed religion inspires him.[33]

In his pursuit of natural history Hitchcock found endless evidence of divine omniscience and felt it his duty to make frequent references of a religious character, but apparently some of them were edited out of his writings for the *Journal*. He wrote to Silliman that 'every remark of a <u>religious</u> character was struck out of the last part of my sketch. . . .' He therefore did not think it was Silliman who had altered a geological sketch in the *Journal*; but, Hitchcock added, he did not mean to complain.[34]

The letters between Hitchcock and Silliman also reflected the deep personal concern they held for one another. In 1821 Hitchcock married Orra White, a former teacher at the Deerfield Academy, and several years later when they lost a child, Silliman tried to comfort the bereaved parents from his own experience.[35]

Always apprehensive about his own health, Hitchcock would inquire anxiously after Silliman's health from time to time, writing in 1821, 'Pray Sir what is your complaint? for I could never learn except that your lungs were affected—That "final release" of which you speak I earnestly pray may be long delayed.'[36] He was sympathetic upon hearing that Silliman was not well, some two years later, 'But from what I learn I have some hope that your constitution is only exhausted—not worn out & that relaxation will recruit it. . . .'[37] The next spring found Silliman better, and Hitchcock recommending the benefits of a bland diet.

> I rejoice to hear of your up hill progress in regard to health. If your complaint is dyspepsia as I learn it is I believe that inferior as I am to you in everything else I could on this point give some instruction as I have had fifteen years of bitter experience. But I shall not attempt to prescribe to an M.D.: yet I must say that some prescriptions of Dr Ives and my bread and milk in the morning have within the year past considerably alleviated my complaints.[38]

Despite his excursions in the outdoors while he was pastor, Hitchcock felt his own health deteriorating, and four years' service, with several revivals, 'brought me into such a state of health that I felt I must get released.'[39] In 1825 Hitchcock was offered the professorship of natural history and chemistry at Amherst College.[40] Once more he sought an opinion from Silliman, who recommended that he accept the position in view of his health and volunteered to send references.[41] Following this advice, Hitchcock resigned the leadership of his congregation, though he was obsessed by the feebleness of his constitution and did not expect to survive long. His letter regarding his decision explained to the church council: 'On consulting judicious persons in various parts of N. England, I found their prevailing opinion to be, that a professorship might be more favourable to my health than the ministry. It seemed then to be an important inquiry with me whether this was not a door opened by Providence for me to be useful a little longer.'[42]

Thus in 1825 began Hitchcock's career as a professor of science. His contributions were to be unique in the history of geology; and as professor and president of Amherst, he guided the college through critical decisions. After thirty-eight years there, he could write in his *Reminiscences*:

> With the 1,520 who have since graduated, I have of course been acquainted, because I have given them all courses of lectures, and heard their recitations in the department assigned me. For I have never been prevented, in any year, from giving my assigned course of instruction, either by sickness or absence. I have also known personally, and as friends, every Instructor who has been connected with the College.[43]

The Amherst historian recorded Hitchcock's first appointment: 'Rev. Edward Hitchcock was chosen professor of chemistry and natural history, with a salary of seven hundred dollars and the privilege of being excused for one year from performing such duties of a professor as he might be unable to perform "on account of his want of full health."' [44]

A strong and modest person, Hitchcock carried to his own students the interest Silliman had shown him; and to his geological and paleontological investigations brought an enthusiasm that had been guided and heightened by Silliman's teaching.

Hitchcock looked forward eagerly to teaching, and soon Silliman was cautioning him that if he undertook all that he was planning '& go on with your usual zeal you will not last long,' and 'as to undertaking a course of chemical demonstrations without a previous apprenticeship in the chemical part, I must say that I think you would meet with much embarrassment. . . .' [45] Hitchcock's *Reminiscences* relate:

> I was dismissed October 25th, 1825, and went to New Haven with Mrs. H., where I stayed till the early part of January, 1826, in the laboratory of Prof. Silliman, by whose kindness and instruction my sojourn there was made most profitable. I there learnt how to perform chemical experiments so that they should rarely fail, and this is the grand secret of success in that department. The two principles for securing success were these, and I had them fixed to the wall of the laboratory:
>
> 1. Never attempt an experiment in public which you have not within a few hours performed in private.
>
> 2. No apology to be ever given or received by any one in the laboratory for a failure, but it is to be set down as detracting so much from the skill of the operator. [46]

Silliman related: 'During this period, and at subsequent times, also, I was aided by private pupils who worked in the Laboratory for the sake of obtaining a knowledge of practical chemistry,' and named Edward Hitchcock as one who was 'among the most distinguished of these.' [47]

Hitchcock was free now to devote himself primarily to science, although the Ecclesiastical Council, in formally dismissing him, had stressed their reluctance to do so except for reasons of his health. 'The council cannot feel themselves justified to dismiss him, for the sake of a professorship at Amherst College or any other literary institution; nor for any other consideration which now occurs to them.' [48]

At the college there was little facility in those early days for the teaching of a chemistry course. Hitchcock recalled, 'When I joined the

College in the winter of 1826, there was no laboratory, no philosophical cabinet, no natural history cabinet, and no chapel.'[49] Two fourth floor rooms in a dormitory were used for lectures in natural philosophy and for the chemistry course, then in the evening for prayer. Hitchcock remembered, 'after I had been manipulating with chlorine,' hearing 'Dr. Humphrey in his introductory petition, apparently unconscious of the odor that was in the room, which the students were snuffling at, pray that the Lord might smell a sweet savor from our offering.'[50]

Hitchcock gave two courses at least in those quarters, then the chapel built in 1826 provided basement space for a chemistry laboratory

> mostly above ground with cellar rooms adjoining. I had ample space for a large lecture room, apparatus room, and office, and means enough were furnished for supplying economically furnaces, cisterns, gasometers and apparatus. The only difficulty was that the room was beneath all the others and partially under ground. But at that time the idea generally was that such was the proper place for the laboratory. Because the chemist eliminates many mephitic gases, therefore place him where he cannot get them out of his room; or if they do escape through the ceiling they will let all in the rooms above him get a whiff of the atmosphere which he is obliged to breathe in concentrated purity. Nevertheless, I spent at least a third of my time for eighteen years in that laboratory, and found it in most respects very convenient.[51]

For many years Hitchcock alone took in charge the teaching of natural history, the subjects of which included: 'Chemistry, Botany, Mineralogy, Geology, Zoölogy, Anatomy and Physiology, Natural Theology'; and sometimes he was temporarily assigned to give instruction in 'Natural Philosophy and Astronomy.'[52] From these beginnings, the historian of Amherst College relates, 'Dr. Hitchcock created the *materiel* and the reputation of Amherst College in the Department of Natural History.'[53]

During this first year of teaching, Hitchcock visited Silliman in New Haven and obtained chemical apparatus and chemicals for his laboratory.[54] By summer 1826 he reported to Silliman: 'I closed my chemical course yesterday—Over the latter part of the subject I hurried rapidly and if Providence permit I hope to attend the last part of your course that I may be better prepared in future.' His experiments had been almost uniformly successful: 'I have reason for thankfulness that I have gone through without receiving scarcely a scratch.'[55]

Visiting Amherst in 1827, Charles Upham Shepard, then Silliman's assistant in the laboratory in New Haven, brought advice on the galvanic apparatus and 'calorimotor.'[56] And Hitchcock eagerly awaited the appearance of Silliman's chemistry text: 'When will you print it? Shall you permit it to be used in other institutions besides Yale?'[57]

When Silliman's book was published, Hitchcock used it for his class. Meanwhile, he continued to receive advice on practical chemistry, and reported in a letter to Silliman: 'P.S. Though I have been blown up once with fulminating silver I shall keep it in phials though in small quantities and uncorked. But I think I must follow your advice.'[58]

He took a personal interest in his students, feeling responsible for their well being at Amherst, both physical and religious. He advised temperance and moderate habits, but confided to Silliman that although 'the most rigid temperance in eating and drinking is doing something for me' and he was 'more comfortable,' it did not restore his 'exhausted stamina.'[59] Hitchcock lectured to the students on diet and regimen, recommending that they avoid intemperance in all forms and advising the pursuit of natural history outdoors for its salutary effects,[60] though as for himself, '. . . it may be that Providence has brought me before you, a living example of the nature and desolating effect of dyspepsy, that you may be roused to flee from the destroyer. . . .'[61]

He was from that time involved with the temperance movement at the college. The *'Antevenean Society* or *the society against poisons'* was founded in 1830, and a large proportion of the students for over thirty years signed pledges of abstinence.[62] In problems of discipline Hitchcock always counted on the force of reason and the gentle suggestion of what was right. Similarly with his dry sense of humor he suggested temperance in an allegorical tract written when he was president—*History of a Zoological Temperance Convention. Held in Central Africa in 1847.* In it he described a meeting of the animals— 'although their language be inarticulate (that is, *without joints*)'[63]—at which one resolution had been

> that this Convention do all in their power to promote the manufacture and the use of alcoholic drinks among men; that the Horse, the Mule, and the Ox, for instance, when called to labor in the wine-press, the cider-mill, or the distillery, cheerfully submit to the severest efforts, because they are taking the most effectual way to prevent the prosperity and increase of their great enemy and persecutor, man.[64]

The explorations that Hitchcock had first undertaken for his health and reported in the initial volume of Silliman's *Journal,* in

'Remarks on the Geology of a Section of Massachusetts on Connecticut River, with a Part of New-Hampshire and Vermont,' had been extended. He had communicated not only on western Massachusetts, but on its eastern reaches in Martha's Vineyard and the Elizabeth Islands. 'I was conversant with the earliest efforts in this country to set up geological surveys,'[65] Hitchcock recalled. When the governor recommended a trigonometric survey of the state to the legislature, Hitchcock suggested a geological survey and was duly appointed the surveyor.[66] In this instance, Silliman described Hitchcock as 'the indefatigable & successful explorer and historian of the geology of Massachusetts, with the liberal aid of that noble State in giving full effect to his labors by furnishing the means of bringing forth with dignity and full illustrations by drawings, maps, sections &c the volumes of reports.'[67]

The preliminary report was reprinted in the *Journal*: 'Report on the Geology of Massachusetts: examined under the direction of the Government of that State, during the years 1830 and 1831,'[68] for Hitchcock hoped to assure the legislature's continued interest in the endeavor and the necessary appropriations.[69] Enlarged and revised in several stages, Hitchcock's reports constituted the state survey 'which has the honor of originating that rapid succession of scientific surveys, which have done so much to develop the mineral and agricultural resources of our country.'[70] After making the first complete report in 1833, Hitchcock wrote to Silliman, who had given his own views in a new edition of Bakewell: 'I shall now hope to get somewhat sheltered behind your arguments and authority for certain heresies which I disclosed in my Report.'[71]

The Massachusetts survey appeared in a second edition in 1835, enlarged, with sections on economical, topographical, and scientific geology, as well as 'Catalogues of Plants and Animals.'[72] It contained a store of information, even an appreciation of the scenery, illustrated by an atlas of drawings executed by Mrs. Hitchcock, who illustrated most of Hitchcock's writings, and was intended to demonstrate not only geological fact but beneficent design. Again Hitchcock discussed the span of geological time, the origin of the Massachusetts diluvium (certainly not Noachian), and the evidence that the Connecticut Valley had once experienced a tropical climate, and 'that this delightful valley, which now forms so charming a residence for man, once constituted, and for an immense period, the bottom of a tropical ocean.'[73] He argued for extinctions and successive creations.

> A careful examination of the fossils of this sandstone, will convince any
> one that their resemblance to any now found living on the globe, is very

faint; so that probably they cannot be referred to in the same genera, much less the same species. This too accords with the facts that have been observed in other parts of the world. The farther down in the series of rocks we penetrate, the more unlike living animals and plants are those found in a fossil state. And it seems to be pretty well established, that there have been several successive creations and extinctions of animals and plants on our globe, before the production of its present organized beings.[74]

Although Hitchcock had been apprehensive about the reception of the conclusions he presented, he saw no challenge to the Mosaic account: 'I find them a striking evidence of the benevolence of the Deity. . . . The globe was evidently preparing for the residence of man, and the other animals that now inherit it.'[75]

Hitchcock kept Benjamin Silliman informed on the progress of the survey and received his support, for such projects were among Silliman's special interests and his former students and assistants made several of the first geological surveys. In addition to the Massachusetts survey—the *Final Report on the Geology of Massachusetts* appeared in 1841—Hitchcock served in 1836 on the New York state survey. But despite his correspondence, Hitchcock felt somewhat isolated and thought that the geologists working on the surveys ought to meet. The American Geological Society, chartered in 1819, in which Hitchcock had participated while he was in New Haven, had long since ceased its activities.[76]

In 1838 Hitchcock suggested to James G. Percival, the state geologist of Connecticut, as he had to Prof. Henry D. Rogers of Philadelphia, 'the desirableness of having a meeting of our geologists especially of those engaged in the surveys in order that they may become better acquainted & present for examination & advice peculiar specimens—difficulties which they may meet.'

He hoped a meeting would be arranged in the near future. Hitchcock wrote, 'I presume that I feel the need of such a meeting more than almost any other rock breaker in the country because I am more insulated.'[77] His suggestion led to the organizational gathering in Philadelphia in 1840 of the Association of American Geologists, at which he was made chairman, and since other geologists besides those engaged in the state surveys attended, Hitchcock related in his *Reminiscences*, 'We added the word "Naturalists" to our name, and appointed Prof. B. Silliman, although never connected with a State survey, Chairman of the next meeting. . . .'[78] 'In 1848 we formally adopted the name of the American Association for the Advancement of Science.' Still another colleague, Prof. H.D. Mather, to whom Hitchcock had written in 1837 and 1838, recollected this origin of the American Association for the Advancement of Science in a letter to Hitchcock: '*You*, so far as I know, first suggested the matter of such an association.'[79]

In 1835 discoveries of large bird-like footmarks in the Connecticut Valley sandstone changed the direction of Hitchcock's scientific investigations. Pliny Moody, as a boy living in South Hadley, had first noticed the footmarks in 1802, but they had been taken for 'tracks of poultry' and given no special notice.[80] An account of the events of 1835 was later sent to the editor of the *American Journal of Science* by Dexter Marsh, who accumulated a great collection of the footmarks along with a description of his many specimens. He had long hesitated, he wrote, 'from reasons unnecessary for me to state, knowing as you do, that I am an unlearned, laboring man.' Marsh reminded him, 'You will recollect that the first specimen of fossil footprints ever brought into public notice in this country, was the slab I discovered among the flagging stone, while laying the sidewalks near my house, which Dr. Deane first described to President Hitchcock as the *footprints of birds*.'[81]

Hitchcock's *Reminiscences* recollect:

> In March, 1835, Mr. W. W. Draper, of Greenfield, walking home from church with his wife noticed on some slabs of flagging stone lying by the sidewalk, impressions which he described to Wm. Wilson, in front of whose house the slabs lay, 'here are some turkey tracks made 3,000 years ago.' Mr. Wilson soon afterward showed them to Dr. Deane, who described them to me by letter the same week, as 'the tracks of a turkey in relief,' and showed a correct appreciation of their nature and value.[82]

The investigation of the fossil footprints in the new red sandstone was to open an era of conjecture and controversy over the nature of the former inhabitants of the Connecticut Valley, for though more and more footprints in the rock were bared, the corresponding fossil remains were not to be found. Silliman recorded in his 'Reminiscences':

> At that time, little was known of the impressions of the feet of birds and animals that have been so fully developed by Dr Deane & Prof Hitchcock. Their researches have given a classical interest to this region which is now renowned wherever geology is cultivated and wherever the records of early life on our globe are studied and appreciated.[83]

Dr. Deane brought the footmarks to Hitchcock's attention, and Hitchcock planned to publish an article in the *Journal* on the impressions, casts of which he sent to Silliman. Hitchcock explained to Silliman:

> My intention is to offer you a paper on this subject for your January No. of the Journal. I shall give to D͟r͟ Deane the credit of having put me on the track after these relics; but I shall hope if consistent you will delay his description until you receive mine as I am sure I shall be able to present a more full and satisfactory view of the case than he can do.

Silliman was to underscore this passage years later on finding this letter and return it to Hitchcock, for a priority dispute in time arose, and he felt it might have been avoided by a clearer acknowledgment of Deane as a 'coworker.'[84] At first it appears to have been satisfactory to Deane that Hitchcock would make the scientific study of the footmarks and present his results, and Hitchcock wrote to him of his presentiment that geologists would not easily accept the evidence that the footprints of birds lay so deep in the strata.[85] Silliman felt the discovery to be valid, and after noting that he expected Deane's role to be recognized, expressed his pleasure that Hitchcock would investigate the tracks. 'It would be a most interesting geological conclusion to establish that there were birds at so early an era as the new red sandstone & especially that turkeys were gobbling & strutting so long before their rival man.'[86]

Soon he was deep in planning for the forthcoming paper, inquiring of Hitchcock, 'Would you wish a plate four foot long or rising, to exhibit the proportionate step as well as the size of the birds' feet. . . .'[87] And a few weeks after: 'I have this day received your drawing of the gigantic birds foot & I am determined it shall appear.'[88] The article was published in 1836 in the *American Journal of Science* with an account of the discovery of the footprints, 'Ornithichnology.—Description of the Foot marks of Birds, (Ornithichnites) on new Red Sandstone in Massachusetts.'

In the meantime Hitchcock was examining a profusion of specimens, which he found nearby: 'In passing over the side walks at Northampton, during the summer, I discovered several examples of similar impressions upon the flagging stones.'[89] He could name a number of localities where the impressions of feet with three toes pointing forward could be seen, and he could group them as varieties, even species.[90] Yet for one species, the evidence indicated great weight. 'Indeed, I hesitate not to say', Hitchcock wrote, 'that the impression made on the mud appears to have been almost as deep, indicating a pressure almost as great, as if an Elephant had passed over it. I could not persuade myself, until the evidence became irresistible, that I was examining merely the track of a bird.'[91] Some of the birds appeared to have had strides of four feet, but this did not surprise Hitchcock, for in the early history of the earth it seemed that temperatures must have been higher and 'favourable to a giant like development of every form of life.'[92]

For several years few scientists besides Silliman and William Buckland defended Hitchcock's views,[93] and he was roundly attacked in the *Knickerbocker* in 1836. Buckland, however, not only quoted Hitchcock and cited his discoveries, but reproduced the astonishing illustrations of the birds' footprints in his *Geology and Mineralogy Considered With Reference to Natural Theology*, also published in 1836 as the sixth of the Bridgewater Treatises. To Buckland, fossil remains that appeared as distinct and ordered species not only demonstrated 'the exercise of stupendous Intelligence and Power,' but 'a chain of connected evidence' of the continuous Being and of the divine Attributes.[94] Hitchcock continued to find and classify new species of the footprints, describing them in his *Final Report*, in the *American Journal of Science*, and elsewhere. In 1841 a report to the Geological Association supported his conclusions on the fossil footmarks.[95]

With the discovery of these fossil tracks, Hitchcock began to gather his famous cabinet, collecting many of his own specimens.

> Whenever I could, I have myself gone to the quarries and dug out the specimens. When not too large, also, I have transported them on my own business wagon. Again and again, have I entered Amherst on such a load, generally, however, preferring not to arrive till evening, because, especially of late, such manual labor is regarded by many as not comporting with the dignity of a professor. I have not, however, in general, paid much attention to such a feeling, except to be pained by seeing it increase, because its prevalence would change the character of the College, by driving away those who are obliged to do their own work.[96]

Other specimens were obtained by purchase, for once the footprints of the Connecticut Valley were recognized, there were eager collectors. One such was Dexter Marsh whom Hitchcock described as the most ambitious of all and whose aim it was 'to get together the largest collection in the world. He succeeded, if we take into account the quality of the specimens. But, poor man! He died before his work was done, having, in my opinion, hastened his decease by excessive labor in the hot sun getting out beryls and other minerals. His executors sold his collections at auction.'[97]

As the footprints became well known, the prices grew higher, Hitchcock noticed, and at auction the bidding rose precipitously.

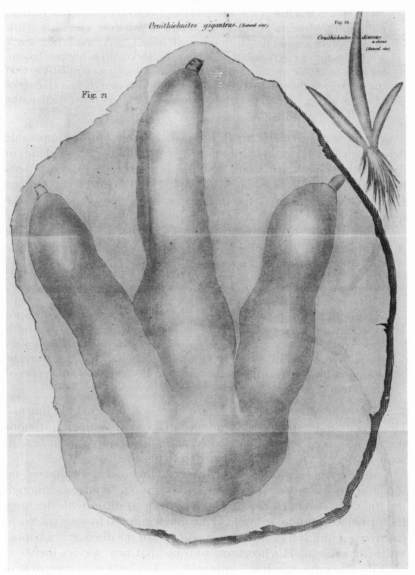

Fig. 21
Ornithichnites giganteus. (Natural size)

Fig. 22
Ornithichnites diversus a clarus (Natural size)

Ornithichnites giganteus. *Fossil footprint in the Connecticut Valley Sandstone, reproduced with Hitchcock's article in the* American Journal of Science, *1836, in its original size, 14½ inches long and 10½ inches wide.*

I found that whenever I expressed any particular interest in a specimen the presumption was that it was rare, and the price went up accordingly. I was obliged, therefore, to exercise a good deal of prudence, and show much *sang froid*, or I could not, with my small means, make much headway. I worked as quietly as possible, with my plans locked up in my own bosom, yet with inflexible resolution and perseverance, looking constantly to God for help. I felt that such a collection would illustrate a curious chapter of His Providence towards our globe, and that the larger the collection, the more full the illustration.[98]

Thus, over years, Hitchcock amassed at Amherst his incomparable 'Ichnological Cabinet' of fossil footprints. Charles Lyell visited him in April 1842[99] and later mentioned the report of the Massachusetts footmarks in his lectures at New York.[100] Silliman, of course, saw Hitchcock's and Deane's specimens at various times, and when the members of the American Association for the Advancement of Science attending the 1859 Springfield meeting took a tour to Amherst, the *American Journal of Science* reported of Hitchcock's cabinet:

> Here Dr. Hitchcock has built up a lasting monument of his original labors in the curious department of foot-marks on the Connecticut sandstone. This vast collection, vast both in the numbers and magnitude of its specimens, is now preserved in 'Appleton Hall,' a new building erected especially for its accommodation, and on the ground floor of which these curious records of lost races once denizens of this lovely valley are spread out to the inspection of visitors. No one can form an adequate notion of the interest of these remarkable collections without a personal inspection.[101]

The year after he first described the footprints in the *Journal*, Hitchcock, in another paper, remarked that certain of the impressions might have been left by four-footed animals, 'some of them bear in some respects so near a resemblance to living Saurians.'[102]

Silliman, meanwhile, was defending Hitchcock's conclusions on the footprints in his correspondence with geologists abroad, although the difficulty remained that the bones of the creatures with the huge footprints were not to be found. 'I am much gratified by your success in discovering bird tracks and hope it will end in the discovery of bones,' Silliman wrote to Hitchcock on hearing that new species had been identified among the fossil prints; '. . . I ache for a comparative anatomist to settle these questions—but—where is he?'[103] Alexandre Brongniart, Gideon Mantell, and Charles Lyell gave the footmarks their attention, and Buckland sent Hitchcock drawings of fossil footprints that had been found in the vicinity of Liverpool.[104] In their letters Hitchcock and Silliman discussed geological opinion, and in one instance disagreed to the point that Hitchcock feared he might have lost Silliman's friendship. Hitchcock was highly critical of Lyell, not for his uniformitarianism—though Hitchcock believed that 'we must admit a far greater intensity in geological agencies in early times than at present' [105]—but because his writings lacked any religious reference: 'If he be a decided believer in Christianity why ~~is he afraid~~ to say so? does he not say so? A single sentence would settle the point— Did anyone ever read the geological writings of Prof. Silliman and doubt whether they were the friends of revelation?' [106]

As he crossed out words, Hitchcock revealed his emotion, but soon Silliman assured him that nothing had disturbed their relationship; [107] subsequently, Hitchcock somewhat modified his feelings about Lyell. After Lyell's visit to New Haven in 1841, Silliman informed Hitchcock, 'M⨦ Lyell spoke very highly of your last report & left his copy here in safe-keeping until he returns from New York State. . . . He will visit you & be most anxious to see the tracks.' [108]

With Hitchcock the next spring, Lyell examined the sites at which the 'Ornithichnites' were to be found. [109] Later Mr. Woods, the benefactor of Amherst College, gave Lyell's opinion of Hitchcock, as Woods '. . . quoted the authority of Mr. Lyell, whom he had heard say that the Doctor knew more of geology and could tell it better than any other man he had met on this side of the Atlantic.' [110]

Meanwhile there was continuing communication among Silliman's circle. Charles Shepard might carry messages, letters, or mineral specimens on his trips between New Haven and Amherst, and sometimes now it was Benjamin Silliman, Jr., who wrote to Hitchcock. In a letter to which his father added a long postscript on Hitchcock's geology, the younger Silliman advised Hitchcock that he had chemicals for him.

> Your kind letter of Oct. 15th by Prof Shepard came safe to hand with its enclosure. . . . I have received from Prof Shepard a box of chemicals for you, similar I presume to one which accompanied it for me. The canal is sealed for this year, & also no doubt the Connecticut river & I write to enquire of you if you wish me to forward it by Stage & RailRoad—very few of the tests are liable to freeze. [111]

The tracks, especially, caught the imagination of all. In the *Final Report* on Massachusetts Hitchcock had grouped the species between 'Sauroidichnites,' resembling those of Saurians or lizards, and 'Ornithoidichnites,' resembling bird tracks, [112] and the estimated size of the creatures that had made the impressions was amazing, judging by the length of the stride: *O. giganteus* had a foot four times as large as that of the African ostrich, the largest living bird; [113] its stride was four to six feet long, and it appeared to have been over twelve feet tall. *O. ingens* might have been eighteen feet high, but Hitchcock was less confident about this measurement. Though there were few fossil remains of their existence, Hitchcock believed that 'the scarcity of organic remains in the new red sandstone, may probably be more owing to something unfavorable to their preservation, than to their not having existed.' And in the former tropical climate, 'from what we know of Divine Benevolence, . . . other gigantic races of animals participated in its blessings.' Hitchcock surmised a rich vegetation as well.[114] Since it was topical, Benjamin Silliman, Jr. sent Hitchcock a poem that a tutor had written in 1837, . . . 'Mr Dana before leaving this country—composed the music . . . & I send you the words & have no doubt but Mr D will furnish the music—if you care to see it—perhaps Miss Hitchcock may play on an instrument.' The poem read:

> When first large birds did walk abroad
>   On rocks but lately cleft
> Proceeding on no beaten road
>   With toes turned right & left:
> What wondrous footsteps left they then
>   Behind them as they stalked
> Ere on this mundane earth or men,
>   or cattle yet had walked.
>
> 2. Full eighteen feet they raised high
>   Their heads into the air
> And Lizard 'Possum Kangaroo
>   Did wag their heads and stare,
> The little fishes were afraid
>   They should be caught for food
> And out into a deeper tide
>   Did swim full many a rood.
>
> 3 Could but our modern eyes behold
>   Those birds of olden time
> Yet marching on their tide washed way
>   With strides full six feet nine
> What trembling joy the heart would fill
>   What gladsome tears the eyes.
> Geologists would not sit still
>   They'd throw their caps on high.

4. Let then each one that looks upon
    The tracks of such a bird
Impressed in sand now turned to stone
    As cheese is made from curd
Reflect if fowls were larger then
    Than fowls that now appear,
Much more their year must
    Sure have been
Far longer than our year

Chorus—
    No Birds like those great birds of Old
    One half the story's not yet told
    About those giant Birds of Old.

The letter closed with a warmly humorous note,

As this was an extempore at dinner table, quite an impromptu—the music
is much better, Mr Dana felt some delicacy on my sending the above to you
but you might think it disrespectful in a stranger to have done so.
                    With much respect,
                        Your friend,
                        B. Silliman, Jr.[115]

Whether the footprints were indeed those of birds remained in
conjecture, even for the two-footed animals. The *Final Report* had
cited Richard Owen's opinion that the evidence was insufficient to
establish that they were birds, for they might have been biped saurians.
Nevertheless, it was Hitchcock's opinion that, since these had three toes
like birds, 'if we judge from comparative anatomy alone it seems to me
we must infer they were made by birds.' He was providing for other
possibilities in his nomenclature, as he wrote to his friend, William
Redfield: 'I am not anxious that these tracks should turn out to be those
of birds & by adopting the term Ornithoidichnites (tracks resembling
those of birds) I have provided for any new discoveries.'[116]

By 1848 he distinguished some that seemed to be the tracks of
birds, others that might have been; lizards and batrachians, and other
forms of animals as well, had left footmarks. Hitchcock had found
forty-nine species, some quadruped, that had left their imprints as they
passed over the ground.[117] He gave careful attention to the distinctive
features of the impressions, for, 'the tracks were made by animals,
almost as certainly as if their skeletons were standing before the
observer.'[118] He clearly recognized that not only the reptiles, but the
former birds, were like none living, and differed in more than size.

The classes of animals which seem to have made the fossil footmarks are of all others most easily distinguished by their feet; I mean reptiles and birds. The chief difficulty in the case lies in the fact, that, in the red-sandstone period, some of these animals seem to have differed not a little in their structure from those now living.[119]

Collecting and examining thousands of footmarks, he continued to struggle with the problem, essentially one of classification, and in the summer of 1855 wrote to Silliman: 'I do not give up the idea that some of our tracks are those of birds. The grand argument for such an opinion still remains untouched: in the number of phalangeal impressions which corresponds with that of birds alone.'[120]

Silliman, too, was reluctant to decide that some of the prints were not those of birds, though Hitchcock had found that certain of the birdlike animals seemed to have made caudal impressions as well as footmarks. Silliman protested: 'Need we give up the birds? To my eye many—very many of the impressions appear as indubitably ornith—as tracks of indubitable living birds made yesterday in clay or sand. . . .'[121]

The next year (1856) an article by Hitchcock in the *American Journal of Science* described new and extraordinary footmarks: 'Upon the whole the evidence is very strong that this animal was an enormous biped with a very long tail!' Once again he raised the possibility, '. . . already repeatedly hinted at by me in former descriptions of footmarks, that many of these extinct animals may have belonged to a type of animal existence intermediate between that of birds and the lower classes of vertebrates.'[122]

In 1858 Hitchcock published his comprehensive *Ichnology of New England*, in which he listed still more species among the animals whose tracks remained impressed on the Connecticut Valley rock; included were fourteen 'Thick-toed Birds' and seventeen 'Narrow-toed Birds.'[123] Yet he was thinking of some of these as 'wingless birds,' and again posed the supposition that various intermediate forms might once have existed, besides the Ichthyosaurus, Plesiosaurus, and the 'other huge Saurian reptiles' he had described. He still believed that the species with 'ornithic' characters were birds when, in 1863, he reported doubts that the number of phalanges was necessarily the deciding factor after all.[124] He took this position also in his last paper in the *American Journal of Science*: '. . . I cannot hesitate to reckon the biped thick-toed Lithichnozoa as birds; for I see no characters in their tracks that ally them to any other animals. I must consider them not only as birds, but as forming a quite perfect type of birds for sandstone days.'

The Archæopteryx had by then been discovered, and he acceded to Dana's views: 'Doubtless with some peculiarities of structure bringing them into the "comprehensive types" of Dana, but still decidedly birds.'[125]

Hitchcock was still considered the foremost authority on the fossil footmarks of the Connecticut Valley a century later by Richard Swann Lull. The great classes that had made the prints had included salamandrine amphibia and reptiles, many of them dinosaurs, and the 'ornithic' prints had in the main been made by dinosaurs; yet Lull ruled the actual presence of birds a moot point until their fossil remains should be found, though he placed the Archæopteryx many millions of years after the close of Newark time, when such large forms roamed.[126]

In his own time, Hitchcock's preeminence as the discoverer of the footprints was challenged, and he was especially sensitive to Benjamin Silliman's view of his role as their first scientific investigator. A priority dispute arose between Deane and Hitchcock; claims and rebuttals appeared in the *American Journal of Science*, where Silliman tried to give fair recognition to both men without hurting Hitchcock's feelings. The pages of the *Journal* had carried the first report of the footprints, and as he tried to limit the duration of the argument, Silliman deplored the use of the *Journal* for a dispute.

Though there had originally been no problem as to who was the discoverer of the footprints, Deane had by now become well informed on their significance. He had studied the footprints, and considered himself the discoverer, having brought them to Hitchcock's attention because he understood that they merited investigation. Silliman had not realized in 1842 when he spoke before the Association of American Geologists and Naturalists at Boston that his description of the footmarks as 'so zealously explored by Dr. James Deane of Greenfield, and both explored and described by Prof. Hitchcock,'[127] had been taken amiss by Hitchcock, and for a while Silliman and Hitchcock did not completely heal this misunderstanding.[128] During 1843 and 1844, as articles on the footprints were published in the *Journal*, the letters of both Hitchcock and Silliman reflected their anxieties that the situation be set right. To his friend Redfield, Hitchcock wrote:

> You will see that the journals and newspapers are discussing the question of who is to be regarded as the original discoverer of those tracks? and they have fairly, as they suppose got the laurel (it was not thought worth contending about till the great men of Europe deigned to endorse my views on the subject) from my brow. After they have said all that they wish

however I shall beg leave to say a few words—although with great reluctance on the subject. I would not do it did not the statements that have been made carry the impression that I have done injustice to others.[129]

Letters from Silliman assured Hitchcock that he regarded him as the first investigator of the footprints: '. . . you are on all hands as far as I am informed regarded as the <u>author & founder of the ornithichnology of the earliest bird era</u> & no one can deprive you of this honor.'[130] Silliman again reassured Hitchcock that he would have worded his Boston address differently had he known it would cause him unhappiness, and thought that 'the more ample terms in which you were spoken of in the same sentence covered your claims.' Recalling attacks that had similarly been made on Lyell, Silliman closed his conciliatory letter, 'It is not worth while to say more now; when we meet I may explain myself. <u>Please to recollect that at the next meeting you will lodge at my house.</u>'[131] Meanwhile he had advised Hitchcock, as well as Deane, on their articles and sent each the other's proofs before publication, and he added, to Hitchcock: 'Remember that these suggestions are from your earliest geological friend and one who stood by you from the first in this matter & has never swerved since—take the suggestions for what they are worth.'[132]

The controversy died down for the time, but was revived now and then, especially at the time of Deane's death in 1858, and upon the posthumous publication of his work on the footprints, with its photographic illustrations.[133] Hitchcock in his *Reminiscences* wrote: 'I claimed not that I first found them, but only that I first scientifically investigated and described them. . . . But I never claimed to be the discoverer unless in this sense.'[134] Silliman in his 'Reminiscences' recalled the dispute as one that might have been averted.

The nomenclature for the makers of the footprints presented Hitchcock with new decisions as he found more species and grouped them; he corresponded with James Dwight Dana on the names he should use and their significance.[135] Silliman and Dana had sent him information and sketches on fossil footprints in the Carboniferous rocks of Pennsylvania. Along with the new classification that Hitchcock sent to Dana in January 1845 went a request that he sound out Professor Silliman about having a genus named for him.

I have used the name of only one naturalist—. . . Prof. Silliman—. On account of his early connection with the subject & the correct views he infuses and I should like to show him this mark of my respect & him <u>alone</u>—But I have not hinted the thing to him or anyone else & therefore I trust you will feel free to express your opinion upon it—If you approve will you ascertain whether Prof. S. will object. You will see I have chosen a genus with three species so that if one should fail the genus will remain.

Among those he would also remember below the genus level were other geological friends. The nomenclature included the terms Shepardianus and Lyellianus, also Sillimani.[136]

Hitchcock had meanwhile been offered the presidency of Amherst College. In April 1845 he took office but, as professor of natural theology and geology, continued to teach. His friend Charles Upham Shepard of New Haven became professor of chemistry and natural history. Of Hitchcock's presidency the Amherst *History* records, 'His weight of character and his wise policy *saved the college.*'[137] The debt was erased and new buildings and cabinets were added. Hitchcock gave the college his collection of fossil footmarks, as he had already given his mineralogical, geological, and zoological collections.[138] When ill health led him, in 1847 and 1850, to travel abroad with Mrs. Hitchcock, he met the leaders of geology in England and was treated with kindness and courtesy by Gideon Mantell and Charles Lyell.[139] His duties as president were heavy, and for a time during this period he seems to have lost touch with Benjamin Silliman.

It may have been their friend Shepard who mended whatever rift occurred. One cause of their estrangement evidently was Hitchcock's failure to give Silliman due recognition in his *Religion of Geology and its Connected Sciences* in 1851, for Silliman wrote in his 'Reminiscences,' 'In his work on the relation of Geology to the Bible he forgot to mention the man who, first in this country vindicated the consistency of those two great subjects.' Silliman's marginal note added, 'A frank apology was afterward made for this omission which was the more to be regretted as Prof[r] Hitchcock first heard this subject discussed in the lectures in Yale College.'[140] Silliman's letter to Hitchcock in October of the next year indicates a resumption of their friendship:

To Rev[d] President Hitchcock

dear Sir

Your letter of the 16th was particularly acceptable as it enables me to return to those relations of friendship which it was painful for me to feel had been in danger of being weakened. The courtesies of science and literature & of a friendship of many years required, as I thought a mention of earlier labors by one who was the first to attempt in this country, to impart instruction in geology, on any considerable scale of effort—and also to meet the difficulties common to all religious minds that had not been enlightened as to the actual structure of the earth.

He pointed to his own and Hitchcock's contributions to the *Journal,* to Hitchcock's investigations, 'which it has ever been my pleasure and pride to set forth in a strong light before my pupils and the public,' and to his own well-known views 'on the question of time in geology.'

> It seemed to me impossible that they should not have recurred to the mind of my earliest pupil and I was therefore fearful that if our friendly relations had not died out, my views were not deemed important enough to be noticed; and still this conclusion was so inconsistent with the demonstrations at Amherst in June 1848 [both Sillimans had attended the dedication of a new cabinet and observatory then], that I was greatly perplexed & then mentioned the subject to our common friend Prof Shepard. I am glad that I broke silence, because the communication has elicited from you a letter conceived in a spirit of Christian and gentlemanly courtesy and I therefore dismiss all feelings of distrust and you will consider this letter as a full recognition of our former friendly relations.

From his own responsibilities on the *Journal,* Silliman could sympathize with the cares Hitchcock had carried as president. The letter continued:

> All that is passed by, that tended to disturb our harmony, we will give to the winds. As to intermission of letters there is quite as much occasion for apology on my part as on yours. I can fully appreciate the nervous burden of your correspondence; believe that not less than 1000 letters a year were written here previous to my relinquishment of the care of the Journal. Now, I am much relieved on that subject and as the evening twilight of life is deepening upon me I am naturally withdrawing from the world and the world from me.[141]

From this time on there were warm exchanges between Silliman and Edward Hitchcock on geology (Hitchcock contributed to the *Journal* in that year) and warm relations between the families including the children. When Hitchcock resigned the presidency in 1854 and returned to his professorship, there was more time for visiting. In the fall of the next year, the Sillimans stayed at the Hitchcocks' home, and Silliman saw the collections of Hitchcock and Shepard at Amherst College. The invitation from Hitchcock had promised a trip to a quarry in South Hadley to see a row of tracks. He hoped that Mrs. Silliman would come, and that they would stay more than one night: 'You know that we live in plain style: but we will try to make you comfortable.'[142]

It was always characteristic of Hitchcock that he held worldly honors in perspective. He had received his own M.A. from Yale as an honorary degree because his health had not allowed him to study for his bachelor's degree as he had planned. Though Hitchcock won distinction as an educator and geologist—he received the LL.D. from Harvard in 1840, the D.D. from Middlebury in 1846—he reflected his own modesty in the humorous little volume he wrote on temperance. In it, at the animals' temperance convention, 'Mr Equus Asinus,' the ass, discussed a proposition to introduce honorary titles among animals:

> He told them that among men it was quite customary to confer honorary titles upon those who had distinguished themselves in any way; and also upon some, who, as it seemed to him, had not distinguished themselves much. These honors were of three kinds: civil, military, and literary. The first two were mainly bestowed by the government; the latter by Literary Institutions. Men considered it a high honor and gratification to receive these distinctions, and to be greeted as General, Colonel, Captain, Honorable, Reverend, Doctor, &c., and he could not doubt that it would be equally pleasant and useful to the animals. The only difficulty would be in discriminating the individuals who were most deserving. He found, upon inquiry among men, that rulers and guardians of Literary Institutions dispensed these honors to four classes of persons: First, to those who deserved them very much by eminent services; Secondly, to those who wanted them very much; Thirdly to those whose enmity was much feared, or whose friendship was very much desired; and Fourthly, to those who needed such honors very much to supply natural deficiencies. . . .[143]

Looking back over his years at Amherst, Hitchcock took satisfaction instead in the 'religious history' of the college, though his own long-held plan to write a major work on natural theology had never been realized; 'all that I have written was but the scaffolding and a few of the braces and pins of the edifice I had hoped to build.'[144] He had kept before him the initial object of the founding of the college: '. . . the education of pious indigent young men,'[145] a classical education, after which many graduates would choose to enter the ministry. A number of revivals took place while he was at Amherst, and as president, he opened his study at certain times for short periods of 'prayer and religious conference.' By his count, almost half of the graduates had become ministers, and more than half when he included clerical teachers.[146]

It was with their religious applications in mind that Hitchcock had built up the cabinets, for the scholar needed collections for his special interests. To defend the tenets of his religion, he

> . . . must see and examine rocks and fossils before he can understand the discussions raised by geology on the age of the world, on the eternity of matter, on the preadamic existence of suffering and death, on special Divine interventions in nature, and on the extent of the deluge. He must study animals and plants, or he cannot refute the advocates of the development hypothesis or the plurality of origin of the human species. Where else but in a college can those who mean to be ministers of the Gospel acquire such knowledge? [147]

These words in his *Reminiscences* in 1863 indicate some of the opinions Hitchcock held on questions of the day in regard to species, several years after the publication of Darwin's work on evolution by means of natural selection. In *The Religion of Geology* he had argued for the great age of the globe and long days of creation, for separate creations (there had been at least six), and several centers of creation from which the animals had migrated. In general, he had held to progressive development, though there were degradations of species, and above all he held that nature maintained a separation of species which confuted hypotheses of transmutation. [148] Throughout the following years in sermons and articles he reiterated his views, especially his belief that the creation of man, like earlier creations, had been through divine agency; that man represented a divine intervention, '. . . a being introduced all at once, superior somewhat in organic structure to the other animals, but raised immeasurably above them all, by his lofty intellectual and moral powers.' [149] He was disturbed by Agassiz's views on species—a threat to religion as he wrote to Dana:

> Since reading your paper on species I have wanted to drop a word in your ear. I have been greatly troubled to find how powerful is the opinion advanced by our friend Prof. Agassiz to the plurality of the species of man upon religion especially upon young men. Multitudes adopt his views & take shelter under his great name & feel that smaller men must not open their mouths. . . . I think religion suffers far more in this quarter than from geological difficulties.

Dana, he believed, was the one to deal with this problem. [150] Hitchcock was not one to change his views markedly on such matters, and if he had, he would still have found room for a benevolent Deity.

His opposition to natural selection is apparent in a remark in his *Reminiscences* on the African gorilla in the Amherst cabinet:

> No other cabinet in this country, at this date, is so largely represented by specimens of this animal. It being the nearest approach of the animals to

man, these specimens have attracted great interest, particularly as they so clearly show the falsity of the notion that the gorilla could ever have changed into man by the 'law of selection.'[151]

Rejecting the theory that a species might pass by insensible degrees into another, Hitchcock maintained that 'history so far does not authorize the conclusion that a law of nature is dropping out some species and introducing others, so as finally to change the whole'; and in any event, man could only have been introduced by a Divine Creator.[152]

As state geologist of Vermont, Hitchcock had meanwhile, in 1861, completed the survey of that state. He was aided in this by his sons, Charles (who was to be state geologist of Maine and to survey New Hampshire), later professor of mineralogy and geology at Dartmouth,[153] and Edward, who became a professor at Amherst. When Hitchcock finished the survey, he turned to his *Reminiscences*, for, as always, he had the premonition that he was not long for this earth. It was said of Hitchcock that 'throughout his entire public life he preached and taught as a dying man. . . .'[154] He closed his *Reminiscences* in 1863. In failing health, his six children grown, and his wife in a last illness, he wrote to Silliman, his lifelong friend:

Dear Sir,
When I opened your letter my eye fell first upon the photograph & it is very perfect & gives the expression of your face like what it was when more than forty years ago I first heard you lecture & a hundred times afterwards so that a crowd of reminiscences came over me and I had quite a crying spell before reading the letter. This shows the weakness of my nerves; but it also shows how powerful was the influence of your eloquence & your kindness upon me in those early days when I was bashful & uncultivated, poor & without scientific friends. Certain it is that your instructions & encouragement & example have had more influence upon me than those of any other man & if I have not been grateful God forgive me!
We have both as you say had interesting fields of labor yours much the widest & most important: mine was [?] & rougher but still opening opportunities for doing good.[155]

Silliman's 'Personal Notices' marked Hitchcock's passing in the winter of 1864: 'A telegram from his son informed me of this painful event—long expected however as his health has been declining—His age was I believe 70. This death took place in the morning of Saturday Feby 27—Funeral on Wedy Mar 2. I was invited by Prest Stearns—but declined the exposure in the winter.'[156]

Hitchcock's contributions as a geologist were widely noted; he was known for his theories on the drift, on the origin of terraces and deltas, and especially for his writings on surface geology.[157] He had combined theological study with attendance at Silliman's lectures on geology, and later as minister, geologist, and educator, had combined science and religion as the deep concerns of his life. As Professor Tyler described him in his memoriam, 'It was his mission to illustrate, in his life as well as by his tongue and pen, the beauty and harmony of the connection between science and religion.'[158]

The closing advice in Hitchcock's *Reminiscences* sent his reader to study geology:

> In the height of balmy summer then, when nature cries out for a respite from protracted cares and labors, let me exhort you to go forth, not with fishing tackle and fowling-piece, (the meagre resort of many,) but with minds well stored with scientific principles, a hammer in hand, and an aneroid barometer by your side, and laying your course for the mountains, learn the character of the rocks, their origin and fossil contents, and seek the evidences of those stupendous revolutions which they have undergone, not forgetting to trace the Divine Hand in them all.[159]

NOTES

[1] Silliman, 'Reminiscences,' V, 89, Silliman Family Papers.

[2] *Ibid.*, V, 17.

[3] *Ibid.*, V, 16.

[4] Silliman to Hitchcock, 24 August 1817, Hitchcock Papers.

[5] Hitchcock to Silliman, 1 September 1817, Hitchcock Papers.

[6] Silliman to Hitchcock, 6 October 1817, Hitchcock Papers.

[7] Silliman to Hitchcock, 27 October 1817, Hitchcock Papers.

[8] Silliman, 'Reminiscences,' V, 17.

[9] Tyler, *Discourse . . . at the Funeral*, pp. 16–17.

[10] Hitchcock, *Reminiscences*, p. 282.

[11] *Ibid.*, p. 284.

[12] *Ibid.*, pp. 310–314.

[13] *Ibid.*, p. 283.

[14] *Ibid.*, p. 285.

[15] *Ibid.*, p. 286.

[16] Hitchcock to Silliman, 6 July 1818, Hitchcock Papers.

[17] Hitchcock to Silliman, 28 September 1818, Hitchcock Papers.

[18] Fisher, *Silliman*, I, 135.

[19] Silliman to Hitchcock, 6 February 1819, Hitchcock Papers.

[20] Hitchcock Papers.

[21] Silliman to Hitchcock, 18 August 1820, Hitchcock Papers.

[22] Silliman, 'Reminiscences,' I, 13, Silliman Family Papers.

[23] Silliman, 'Introductory Remarks,' *Am. J. Sci.*, 1818, *1*, 8.

[24] Hitchcock, *Reminiscences*, p. 287.

[25] Hitchcock to Silliman, 9 April 1821, Hitchcock Papers. See also 'Fossil Fish,' *Am. J. Sci.*, 1821, *3*, 365-366.

[26] Hitchcock to Silliman, 1 December 1822, Hitchcock Papers.

[27] Hitchcock to Silliman, 6 August 1821, Hitchcock Papers.

[28] Hitchcock, *Utility of Natural History*.

[29] Hitchcock to Silliman, 25 November 1823, Hitchcock Papers.

[30] Hitchcock to Silliman, 20 October 1823, Hitchcock Papers.

[31] Hitchcock, *Utility of Natural History*, p. 24.

[32] *Ibid.*, pp. 26-27.

[33] *Ibid.*, p. 28.

[34] Hitchcock to Silliman, 17 December 1823, Hitchcock Papers.

[35] Silliman to Hitchcock, 20 March 1824, Hitchcock Papers.

[36] Hitchcock to Silliman, 6 August 1821, Hitchcock Papers.

[37] Hitchcock to Silliman, 20 October 1823, Hitchcock Papers.

[38] Hitchcock to Silliman, 21 March 1824, Hitchcock Papers.

[39] Hitchcock, *Reminiscences*, p. 287.

[40] Tyler, *History of Amherst College During its First Half Century*, p. 160.

[41] Silliman to Hitchcock, 14 April 1825, Hitchcock Papers.

[42] Hitchcock Papers.

[43] Hitchcock, *Reminiscences*, Preface [p. v].

[44] Tyler, *History of Amherst College During its First Half Century*, p. 154.

[45] Silliman to Hitchcock, 27 July 1825, Hitchcock Papers.

[46] Hitchcock, *Reminiscences*, p. 288.

[47] Silliman, 'Reminiscences,' V, 10, Silliman Family Papers.

[48] Papers of Rev. Edward Hitchcock relating to the Pastorate at Conway, Hitchcock Papers.

[49] Hitchcock, *Reminiscences*, p. 288.

[50] *Ibid.*, pp. 288-289.

[51] *Ibid.*, p. 73.

[52] Tyler, *Discourse . . . at the Funeral*, p. 24.

[53] *Ibid.*, p. 25.

[54] See letters of Hitchcock to Silliman, 21 March and 18 April 1826, Hitchcock Papers.

[55] Hitchcock to Silliman, 8 July 1826, Hitchcock Papers.

[56] Hitchcock to Silliman, 30 December 1827, Hitchcock Papers.

[57] Hitchcock to Silliman, 7 August 1828, Hitchcock Papers.

[58] Hitchcock to Silliman, 4 March 1832, Hitchcock Papers.

[59] Hitchcock to Silliman, 24 January 1830, Hitchcock Papers

[60] Hitchcock, *Dyspepsy*, p. 233.

[61] *Ibid.*, p. 359.

[62] Hitchcock, *Reminiscences*, p. 152.

[63] Hitchcock, *History of a Zoological Temperance Convention*, [p. 13].

[64] *Ibid.*, p. 147.

[65] Hitchcock, *Reminiscences*, p. 363.

[66] *Ibid.*, pp. 364–365.

[67] Silliman, 'Reminiscences,' V, 17, Silliman Family Papers.

[68] *Am. J. Sci.*, 1832, 22, 1–69.

[69] Hitchcock to Silliman, 4 March 1832, Hitchcock Papers.

[70] Tyler, *Discourse . . . at the Funeral*, p. 23.

[71] Hitchcock to Silliman, 30 December 1833, Hitchcock Papers.

[72] Hitchcock, *Report on the Geology . . . of Massachusetts*.

[73] *Ibid.*, p. 246.

[74] *Ibid.*, p. 247.

[75] *Ibid.*, pp. 249–250.

[76] Silliman, 'Reminiscences,' IV, 92, Silliman Family Papers.

[77] Hitchcock to Percival, 10 April 1838, Percival Papers.

[78] Hitchcock, *Reminiscences*, p. 369.

[79] *Ibid.*, p. 371.

[80] *Ibid.*, pp. 86–87.

[81] Dexter Marsh, 'Fossil Footprints,' *Am. J. Sci.*, 1848, *2nd ser. 6*, 272.

[82] Hitchcock, *Reminiscences*, p. 82.

[83] Silliman, 'Reminiscences,' IV, 97, Silliman Family Papers.

[84] Hitchcock to Silliman, 30 July 1835, with annotation by Silliman to Hitchcock, 19 September 1846, Hitchcock Papers. Silliman, 'Reminiscences,' V, 18 vis., Silliman Family Papers.

[85] Extract of letter, Hitchcock to Deane, 21 September [1835], Hitchcock Papers.

[86] Silliman to Hitchcock, 6 August 1835, Hitchcock Papers.

[87] Silliman to Hitchcock, 23 November 1835, Hitchcock Papers.

[88] Silliman to Hitchcock, 11 December 1835, Hitchcock Papers.

[89] *Am. J. Sci.*, 1836, *29*, 308.

[90] *Ibid.*, pp. 315–316.

[91] *Ibid.*, p. 319.

[92] *Ibid.*, pp. 332–333.

[93] Hitchcock, *Reminiscences*, p. 87.

[94] Buckland, *Geology and Mineralogy*, I, viii, 86.

[95] Hitchcock, *Final Report on the Geology of Massachusetts*, pp. 2a–3a.

[96] Hitchcock, *Reminiscences*, pp. 84–85.

[97] *Ibid.*, pp. 81–82.

[98] *Ibid.*, p. 84.

[99] Lyell, *Travels in North America*, I, 251.

[100] Lyell, *Eight Lectures on Geology*, p. 39.

[101] 'The Thirteenth Meeting of the American Association for the Advancement of Science,' *Am. J. Sci.*, 1859, 2nd ser. *28*, 293.

[102] Edward Hitchcock, 'Fossil Footsteps in Sandstone and Graywacke,' *Am. J. Sci.*, 1837, *32*, 174–176.

[103] Silliman to Hitchcock, 7 November 1836, Hitchcock Papers.

[104] Hitchcock to Redfield, 4 April 1839, Redfield Papers.

[105] Hitchcock, *Elementary Geology*, p. 254.

[106] Hitchcock to Silliman, 12 March 1837, Hitchcock Papers.

[107] Silliman to Hitchcock, 17 March 1837, Hitchcock Papers.

[108] Silliman to Hitchcock, 23 September 1841, Hitchcock Papers.

[109] Charles Lyell, 'On the Fossil Foot-prints of Birds and Impressions of Rain-drops in the Valley of the Connecticut,' *Am. J. Sci.*, 1843, *45*, 393–397.

[110] Tyler, *History of Amherst College During its First Half Century*, p. 317.

[111] Silliman, Jr., to Hitchcock, 7 December 1840, Hitchcock Papers.

[112] Hitchcock, *Final Report on the Geology of Massachusetts*, p. 476.

[113] *Ibid.*, p. 522.

[114] *Ibid.*, pp. 523–524.

[115] Silliman, Jr., to Hitchcock, 11 August 1842, Hitchcock Papers.

[116] Hitchcock to Redfield, 21 November 1842, Redfield Papers.

[117] Edward Hitchcock, 'An Attempt to discriminate and describe the Animals that made the Fossil Footmarks of the United States and especially of New England,' *Mem. Am. Acad. Arts Sci.*, 1848, 2nd ser. *3*, 131.

[118] *Ibid.*, p. 135.

[119] *Ibid.*, p. 137.

[120] Hitchcock to Silliman, 19 August 1855, Hitchcock Papers.

[121] Silliman to Hitchcock, probably late 1855, Hitchcock Papers.

[122] Edward Hitchcock, 'On a new Fossil Fish, and new Fossil Footmarks,' *Am. J. Sci.,* 1856, *2nd ser. 21,* 99.

[123] Hitchcock, *Ichnology of New England,* pp. 178–179.

[124] Hitchcock, *Supplement . . . Ichnology of New England,* pp. 31–33.

[125] Edward Hitchcock, 'New Facts and Conclusions respecting the Fossil Footmarks of the Connecticut Valley,' *Am. J. Sci.,* 1863, *2nd ser. 36,* 55.

[126] Lull, *Triassic Life,* pp. 26, 147.

[127] Silliman, 'Address before the Association of American Geologists Assembled at Boston, April 24, 1842,' *Am. J. Sci.,* 1842, *43,* 241.

[128] Silliman to Hitchcock, 19 September and 19 December 1844, Hitchcock Papers.

[129] Hitchcock to Redfield, 10 August 1843, Redfield Papers.

[130] Silliman to Hitchcock, 13 September 1843, Hitchcock Papers.

[131] Silliman to Hitchcock, 1 November 1844, Hitchcock Papers.

[132] Silliman to Hitchcock, 10 August 1844, Hitchcock Papers.

[133] Deane, *Ichnographs.*

[134] Hitchcock, *Reminiscences,* p. 86.

[135] Hitchcock to J. D. Dana, 1 January 1845, Dana Family Papers.

[136] Hitchcock to Dana, 27 January 1845, Dana Family Papers.

[137] Tyler, *History of Amherst College During its First Half Century,* p. 359.

[138] *Ibid.,* p. 328.

[139] Hitchcock, *Reminiscences,* pp. 337–341, 347–348.

[140] Silliman, 'Reminiscences,' V, 18.

[141] Silliman to Hitchcock, 27 October 1852, Hitchcock Papers.

[142] Hitchcock to Silliman, 20 September 1855, Hitchcock Papers. See also Silliman, 'Personal Notices,' XVI, 6, 8 October 1855, Silliman Family Papers.

[143] Hitchcock, *History of a Zoological Temperance Convention,* pp. 141–142.

[144] Hitchcock, *Reminiscences,* p. 392.

[145] *Ibid.,* p. 2.

[146] *Ibid.,* pp. 160–167, 188, 190–191.

[147] *Ibid.,* p. 113.

[148] Hitchcock, *Religion of Geology,* pp. 24, 64, 70, 165–166, 171, 312, 314, 318–319.

[149] Hitchcock, 'Special Divine Interpositions in Nature,' *Biblthca sacra,* 1854, *11,* 793.

[150] Hitchcock to Dana, 4 July 1858, Dana Family Papers.

[151] Hitchcock, *Reminiscences,* p. 95.

[152] Edward Hitchcock, 'The Law of Nature's Constancy Subordinate to the Higher Law of Change,' *Biblthca sacra,* 1863, *20,* 510.

[153] *Dictionary of American Biography,* s.v. 'Hitchcock, Charles Henry.'

[154] Tyler, *Discourse . . . at the Funeral,* p. 45.

155 Hitchcock to Silliman, 7 May 1863, Hitchcock Papers.

156 Silliman, 'Personal Notices,' XVII, 327, Silliman Family Papers.

157 Merrill, *Contributions*, pp. 367-368, 393-394, 462-463, 510-511.

158 Tyler, *Discourse . . . at the Funeral*, p. 15.

159 Hitchcock, *Reminiscences*, p. 406. Examination of the oil portrait of Hitchcock will show that he is holding in hand an aneroid barometer used by geologists and surveyors, especially on mountains.

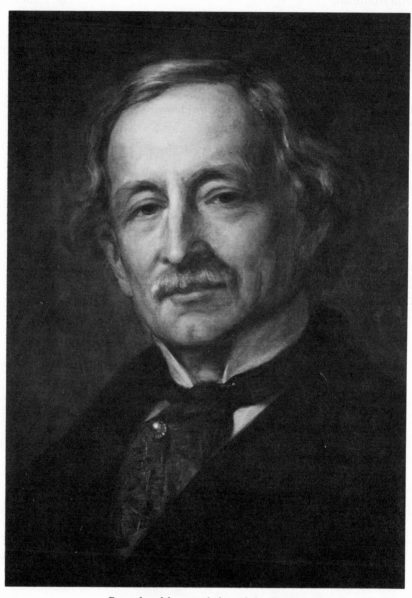

Charles Upham Shepard, artist unknown.

Charles Upham Shepard

GLORIA ROBINSON

IN HIS 'REMINISCENCES' under the heading *Results in Life in regard to my regular assistants [who] Became Professors of Science,* Benjamin Silliman listed Charles Upham Shepard.[1] Shepard's teaching—in mineralogy, chemistry, and various fields of natural history at Yale and at Amherst, and as professor of chemistry at the Medical College of South Carolina—carried many of Silliman's enthusiasms to still another generation of students. As an undergraduate at Amherst, then from Silliman's own chemistry laboratory, often in later years from Charleston, Shepard contributed to the *American Journal of Science,* reporting new mineral localities, and describing and analyzing new mineral species and meteoric specimens.

Shepard was a collector whose vast cabinets, amassed throughout his lifetime, were among the splendors of the day. Long afterwards he recalled Silliman's kindly support of his studies when he first came to New Haven and before he had become Silliman's assistant.

> He manifested the deepest interest in favoring and assisting me in all my studies, permitting me to examine freely the treasures of the Gibbs Cabinet of Minerals, then the only one of note in the country,—and encouraged me to engage in chemical researches, accompanied by the generous permission of ordering for the Laboratory whatever might be needed in their prosecution.[2]

For the use of manuscript sources, I am indebted to the Yale University Library; the Beinecke Rare Book and Manuscript Library, Yale University; and the Amherst College Library. All quotations from the Charles Upham Shepard Papers, The President Edward Hitchcock Papers, and the *Amherst Graduates' Quarterly* are made with the permission of the Trustees of Amherst College, as is the reproduction of the oil portrait of Charles Upham Shepard. I thank J. Richard Phillips and Diana Brown for many kindnesses during my researches in the Special Collections at the Amherst College Library, and Judith Schiff for her help in the use of the Silliman Family Papers in the Manuscripts and Archives of the Yale University Library. Lewis A. Shepard made possible the inclusion of the painting of Charles Upham Shepard from the Amherst collection.

I am especially grateful to the late Dr. Joseph I. Waring for making available the resources of the Waring Historical Library at the Medical University of South Carolina in response to my inquiries, and to Anne Donato for searching this library and further sources in Charleston for newspaper articles, minutes of the Faculty of the Medical College, and other material. The South Caroliniana Library, University of South Carolina, and Mrs. Heard Robertson permitted publication from original letters.

Visiting Amherst in 1855, Silliman remarked in his 'Personal Notices': 'Prof Shepard's cabinet of minerals is very rich especially in gems and meteorites including meteoric iron. In this department it has no equal except in the Imperial Cabinet of Vienna.'[3]

Silliman might likewise have taken pride in having recommended Shepard for appointment to the faculty of the Medical College of South Carolina: '. . . and being appealed to from Charleston regarding the merits of M<u>r</u> Shepard I gave an opinion decidedly in his favor.'[4] Shepard, in his turn, taught chemistry to a host of students, and a Charleston memoriam in 1886 marked his influence: 'Indeed, it has been said that there are very few physicians of advanced age in the Southern States who do not trace their success to the teaching of their revered and beloved Prof. Shepard.'[5]

Shepard's admiration of Silliman stemmed from his reading, as a boy in Rhode Island, Silliman's *Journal of Travels*. 'The perusal of the work imparted a color to my entire existence. And although nearly twenty years elapsed before I met with the author, and not until many years after the death of my father, as soon as I saw him, my heart went out to meet him with the feelings of a son.'[6]

As a schoolboy Shepard began the collections which were to be his lifelong joy: 'My Mineralogical Cabinet was commenced at the age of fifteen, while a member of the Providence Grammar School. . . .'[7] He entered Brown University, but after a year, upon the death of his father (the Reverend Mase Shepard of Tiverton), his mother (Deborah Haskins Shepard) moved with her children to Amherst. He then transferred to the new college in that town.[8] He visited localities where tourmalines and other minerals were to be found and traded his duplicates with the Austrian Consul-General for foreign mineral specimens.[9] At that time Amherst College had little material for illustration of the scientific courses, and President Hitchcock wrote in his *Reminiscences*, of Shepard and his early cabinet, that, '. . . being in a new and unexplored region he was stimulated to search out its mineral and botanical riches. Instead of finding collections at Amherst to study, his own furnished Professor Eaton with the means of lecturing.'[10]

While still a student, Shepard sent communications to Silliman for the *Journal*. After graduating in 1824, Shepard, at the age of twenty, went to Cambridge to study botany and mineralogy under Thomas Nuttall,[11] but his continuing correspondence with Silliman led him to ask to study in Silliman's laboratory. He had spent some months there when Silliman offered him the position as his assistant, succeeding Dr. Noyes and upon the latter's recommendation.[12]

Silliman recorded his favorable impression of the young assistant.

Charles Upham Shepard This gentleman had been for a year or more
residing in New Haven as a student of Natural Science. He had brought
with him a reputation for the love of science especially of Mineralogy and
Chemistry and he had given lectures at some of the schools in Boston. His
manners were amiable and gentlemanly and moral character pure. He was
not an alumnus of Yale College but of Amherst. . . . Mr Shepard was
already proficient in Mineralogy, and his services were at this time
particularly acceptable in that department as I was now to resume the
lectures in the cabinet which had been suspended or imperfectly given of
late.

He was also, to a considerable extent, acquainted with geology, and was
advancing in both of these departments. He had formed habits of travelling to observe localities of minerals, fossils &c and his views were directed
to science as the business of life.[13]

Assisting the professor of chemistry in preparing the lecture
demonstrations was an experience so exciting that Shepard could
describe the scenes of the experiments years afterward as though they
were still before his eyes.

I found myself introduced at once to an engrossing charge. The Professor
fairly reveled in experiments; and these must never fail,—it being the
maxim of the laboratory, that performance was better than apology,
however adroitly made, and an absolute rule, that nothing capable of
visual representation should be omitted. During the lecture hour there was
no lull or intermission; all was rapid movement, a constant appeal to the
delighted senses. Here were broad irradiations of emerald phosphores-
cence, there the vivid spangles of burning iron, or the blinding effulgence
of the compound blow-pipe, or the galvanic deflagrator. Strange sounds
saluted the ear, from the singing hydrogen tube, the crackling decrepita-
tion up to the loud explosions of mingled gases and detonating fulmi-
nates. As forms of matter once regarded simple were torn into their
elements, or these again compounded in manifold ways, a very kaleido-
scope of changes came into view, of which the greatest was the transforma-
tion of the whole seeming fantasy into science, through the lucid rationale
of the gifted lecturer.[14]

A strong personal tie grew up when Shepard became engaged to
Harriet Taylor, an adoptive daughter of the Sillimans. Silliman's
'Personal Notices' relate:

Mrs Shepard was Harriet Taylor, daughter of a merchant in Boston and
both her parents died when she was but little beyond infancy. She came to
Mrs Apthorp's school in New Haven being previously engaged to M^r

Shepard who in 1826 became my assistant in the Laboratory and remained so until 1830—.

In 1831 they were married when M[r] Shepard having resigned his place with me took charge of the Franklin Institute established by M[r] James Brewster of New Haven.[15]

The marriage reinforced Shepard's filial relationship to Silliman, and as the Shepards always considered New Haven their home, and the families lived near each other, they remained close. Silliman recalled that 'my late excellent wife took the orphan girl under her wing while she was here at school and treated her as a daughter. We have ever regarded them and their children with unvarying affection and active friendship.'[16]

In contrast to the emphasis Silliman placed on the reconciliation of science and religion, Shepard's religious views found little reflection in his scientific work. But his brother George C. Shepard, who became a minister, revealed the anxiety his family felt about Charles's religious status, and their hopes that his fiancée might improve his attitude. Religious belief required more than passive acceptance. Public profession and active conversion were deemed necessary. In March 1830 George wrote that Harriet's letter had given their mother and sisters 'much joy,'

> And now I am upon this subject, I trust you will excuse me, when I say, I hope she will view <u>one</u> point of duty in a different light from what you have. I mean that of publicly professing her faith in Jesus, and regarding the ordinances of religion. Religion does not consist in a correct belief in its doctrines, and a few happy emotions of the heart, but in <u>obedience</u> to <u>every requirement</u> which He has made who purchased redemption for us.

He hoped 'at least that Harriet will set you a good example.'[17]

Charles Shepard, who seems not to have been converted earlier through any revival such as that experienced by Silliman at Yale, apparently reassured him; and in May George wrote that he had heard from Mrs. Shepard that Charles was going to profess his 'faith in the Saviour.'[18]

Silliman's records note that Shepard assisted him for five years. 'In 1831—I obtained for him the appointment of Lecturer on Botany in Y. College the attendance on these lectures being voluntary.'[19] He also remarked, as Shepard's colleagues and students did throughout the years, on Shepard's pleasant demeanor and good manners: 'His society was congenial and we proceeded in our duties with entire harmony. His manners were habitually polite and respectful and his temper so amiable that during our whole intercourse there was never a moment of irritation, still less of alienation.'[20]

The invitation to head the Franklin Institution of New Haven, at a salary of $1,000, made it possible for Shepard to marry.[21] Resigning his position with Silliman in 1831, he assumed, upon Silliman's recommendation, the direction of this institution dedicated to supplying the citizens of New Haven with '. . . *popular lectures, collections in several departments of natural history, and facilities for obtaining practical information relating to the application of science to the arts.'*[22] Temporarily Shepard lent his cabinet of minerals to the new school,[23] and here again, prepared the experiments when Silliman gave lectures in chemistry 'adapted to the popular mind of both sexes.' Silliman found that '. . . I had therefore little to do, except to review the arrangements which in the experienced hands of Mr Shepard I was sure would be correctly made.' Shepard gave several courses, 'always with ability and success.'[24]

When in 1832 Benjamin Silliman made his 'Investigations of the Culture of the Sugar Cane and the Manufacture of Sugar Crude and refined'[25] for the government, Shepard and Oliver P. Hubbard assisted him. Shepard surveyed areas in several southern states including Louisiana, Florida, and Georgia. According to Silliman's memorandum, 'Mr Shepard will select those plantations and establishments which are reputed to be the most extensive and the best conducted: he will be particular to understand all the processes and see as many of them as possible.'[26]

A letter of introduction in Silliman's hand explained the purpose of Shepard's visits—'for the common benefit of the nation,' and especially for those concerned with sugar production—and vouched for his character.

> I do hereby also cordially recommend Mr Shepard as a gentleman of integrity, honor and fidelity, as a man of science, and as one in every respect worthy of entire confidence.
>
> Yale College, New Haven
> Nov 7, 1832
>
> B. Silliman
> Prof of Chemistry and Agent under the Secretary of the treasury for the purposes above stated.[27]

Meanwhile the Sillimans looked after Mrs. Shepard, and on Christmas Day 1832 Silliman wrote to reassure Shepard, who was then in Mobile, Alabama, that 'Mrs Shepard gets along finely in her housekeeping—I have seen that her wants are supplied for hay and coal.'[28]

Shepard's observations became part of the final report, and Silliman noted that 'the gentlemen associated with me in that enterprise were active and zealous in their efforts, and they received kind and generous aid on the part of the proprietors and manufacturers in the several places they visited.'[29]

Shepard published part one of his *Treatise on Mineralogy* in 1832. The review in the *Journal* noted that it dealt with 'mineralogy as a separate science, separating from it a variety of information formerly belonging to it,' using the methods employed 'in the other branches of Natural History'; for 'the way in which the science has heretofore been treated among us, has obviously lacked the convenience and precision of its sister sciences Botany and Zoology.'[30]

When the second part appeared three years later, the *Treatise* bore a grateful dedication to Silliman.

> The distinguished services you have rendered to the cause of Mineralogy and Geology in America, not merely in contributing to their early introduction, but to their cultivation among us. . . .
>
> The wisdom and zeal of those exertions which secured to Yale College the most splendid collection of minerals in the country, the valuable instruction and enthusiasm imparted by your lectures to a great body of young men now dispersed through the whole nation, and the public spirit which has led you at a personal sacrifice to maintain in the American Journal of Science a free medium for the diffusion of this kind of knowledge. . . .[31]

With a new appointment as lecturer on natural history at Yale in 1833, Shepard's teaching took on broader outlines; he especially enjoyed lecturing on conchology, using his own shell collection and fossil shells for comparison.[32] He continued to assist with the *Journal*, contributing various miscellanies and translations of foreign articles, entering frequent articles of his own on mineralogical subjects, and describing and verifying meteorite specimens. In 1834 the *Journal* announced that he was establishing a '*private school of Mineralogy and other Branches of Natural History*' and predicted its success, '*provided a sufficient number of pupils should attend, to afford a fair compensation to the highly qualified gentleman. . . .*'[33]

Shepard encouraged students who shared his interest in minerals; a note in the *Journal* in 1832 describes one of James Dwight Dana's discoveries while he was still an undergraduate at Yale. 'My attention was called a few weeks ago, by Mr. J. D. Dana of the Junior Class in Yale College, to a small geode of beautifully transparent crystals imbedded in trap, collected by him at a spot, near the village of Middlefield, called Middletown Falls.'[34]

It was Shepard who in 1835 introduced Dana to Benjamin Silliman, who later appointed Dana assistant in the chemistry laboratory.[35] Shepard had recognized Dana's ability, as a letter from Dana to his father, explaining his wish to remain in New Haven, reported excitedly on 13 April 1835:

> As one thing, I refer to my success in obtaining a place in Silliman's *Journal of Science* for an article of mine, that, but for the encouragement of a scientific person here and his entire approval of it, would probably have remained for a long time unpublished. This person was so much pleased with the system exposed in it that he spoke of introducing it into his *Mineralogy* when he publishes a second edition. The first is now nearly ready for sale. You remember that I was writing for several days at home. That subject also has much pleased this same person (Mr. Shepard, formerly assistant to Professor Silliman), and so much so that he has made use of its principles in a catalogue of minerals to be appended to his forthcoming *Mineralogy*. He will, of course, give credit to whom credit is due. He also encourages me in writing on other subjects. . . .[36]

And as Silliman wrote later, 'The proof is before the world that Mr Shepard did not err.'[37]

On his return from lecturing in Nantucket in 1835, Silliman recalled in his 'Reminiscences', the Medical College of South Carolina requested his opinion of Shepard, and that autumn Shepard began teaching chemistry at Charleston,[38] lecturing to the medical students during the colder months and returning to his New Haven home in the spring. The Charleston *News and Courier*, placing Shepard's first association with the medical school in 1834, recounted:

> It was at this time he came to Charleston, an accomplished scholar and a refined and courteous gentleman, and became identified with the South Carolina Medical College. The College was then enjoying an enviable distinction among similar institutions in the United States. It was the pride and boast of the Southern States, and was the resort of students from all parts of the Union; and it was Dr. Shepard's reputation which, in a large measure, sustained the high position which the College held for at least thirty years of its existence.[39]

Silliman's former students and assistants took part in a number of the first state geological surveys. Tirelessly journeying throughout Connecticut in 1835, Shepard, with Dr. James G. Percival, conducted the geological survey that had recently been authorized in the legislative session. The endeavor had actually been proposed more than twenty-five years earlier by Silliman to the Connecticut Academy of Arts and Sciences, but there had never before been funds for this purpose.[40] Percival's report told of their investigations. 'I was invited by Gov. EDWARDS to engage in the geological department of that survey, in connexion with Prof. C. U. SHEPARD, in the mineralogical department. During the summer of that year, I travelled, with Prof. SHEPARD, through every town in the State. . . .'[41] Shepard's report appeared in 1837,[42] and Percival's five years later.

Meanwhile, in his teaching at Charleston, Shepard gave the course in chemistry 'Definition—Connections with natural history and natural philosophy—Physical qualities of elements—Laws of chemical combination.'[43] He set up scientific apparatus and collections; the catalogue of the Medical College for the 1837-38 session gave its advantages and listed among the facilities '. . . an excellent Chemical apparatus; a splendid cabinet of Minerals deposited and arranged by Professor Shepard.'[44]

When the Shepards were in Charleston, letters flowed back and forth between the two families. Silliman, giving Mrs. Silliman 'two blank pages,' wrote, 'We are grateful to hear that you are both well and that your course proves so valuable; I dare say you have helped to enhance its value & I trust it will grow that more lucrative.'[45] Another note from Silliman thanked Shepard for his letters and mentioned the Shepards' small daughter, Harriet Silliman Shepard, continuing, 'You have been very kind in answering so many letters & I must repay you by minding your affairs again next winter.'[46] From Charleston to New Haven, Shepard wrote, 'I believe Mrs. Shepard is trying to find time from the care of the babe to write a letter to Mrs. Silliman which will accompany this. . . ,' and of the chemistry course he reported, '. . . the class numbers 210.'[47]

When Silliman visited Charleston in 1845, the Shepards welcomed him:

Sab. Feb 2 Charleston

Our friend Prof^r Shepard sent down an omnibus and we were soon in our room at Miss Smith's where our friends reside

. . . .

The churches not being warmed I was afraid to sit in one without a fire & remained at home with a good fire in our chamber and appropriate employments. In the afternoon I went with Mrs Shepard to a small Episcopal church to which she resorts because it is warm.[48]

Silliman enjoyed the cordial hospitality of Charleston and attended one of Professor Shepard's lectures 'at the Medical College an ample and well furnished establishment.'

Prof[r] C. U. S. insisted on introducing me to his class who received me with a round of foot applause—repeated again & again & Mr Legare—as I went in whispered to me that I must say something—so I remarked bowing to them on all sides—'Young gentlemen—I am very happy to meet you under the instruction of one whom I know to be equally zealous & capable and I doubt not you are of the same opinion'—applause again & the lecture proceded. It was on chlorides & iodides and was well got up & illustrated. The class about 200—now about 150 numbers having left town. Their appearance was very respectable—only 9 or 10 wore their hat—only one had his legs over the bar of the next seat in front and one of his feet upon the bench. The laboratory is very amply furnished & is a model of that order & neatness for which Prof[r] C.U.S. is so remarkable.[49]

This was the view the professors had of the medical students. A few days before Silliman's visit, one of the students had written in a letter his judgment of Shepard:

Dr. Sheppard (Chemistry) I was much pleased with at first but my liking soon began to diminish and continued to do so until it was merged in dislike and this is constantly increasing. However he is not unpopular with the class. I believe he is a good chemist but he is a bloodthirsty murderer of all elocution pleases himself in an astonishing degree in everything he does & says has the most winning way as I conceive to gain dislike and in short is a genuine specimen of the produce [?] of Connecticut.[50]

Shepard arranged not only mineralogical collections, but botanical facilities as well. Another student's letter describes plants and greenhouses, fragile and somewhat inhibiting the medical students' natural exuberance:

The old campus grounds in which the boys carried on in a noisy and indecorous manner, have been converted into a fairy-land thro' Dr. Shepard's taste and skill and wealth, covered with hot-houses gorgeously appointed to exhibit almost every tropical plant. The very steps of the Institution are occupied by stands and flower-pots with every variety of geraniums. The entire college grounds resemble a floral-fair. Ladies are in the habit of visiting this part of our old city in their vehicles just to take a look at the premises. . . . Of course, such refinement of taste and culture on the part of our colleague, reflected from every point of view within the enclosure, naturally begets a feeling of restraint among those of our pupils, who would vent their natural instincts in pelting each other with bricks or stones, since they are affraid [sic] of smashing Prof. Shepard's glass-houses and demolishing his exotics. Upon physiological principles, therefore, these automatic explosions, which would manifest themselves either in pugilistic encounters, or brick-bat warfare, are diverted into other channels and find escape in electric nerve-currents evoking such nerve force as we term cerebration—that sets the brain, instead of the muscles, working and engenders thoughts concerning what may have been taught in the last lecture.[51]

Distinguished visitors found Shepard a kind host who might show them the college's zoological specimens. Charles Lyell, in *A Second Visit to the United States of North America*, wrote:

> In the museum of the Medical College, Professor Shepard showed me a fine specimen of the large rattle-snake of South Carolina (Crotalus adamantinus), preserved in spirits. It was said to have been nine years old, having six rattles, the tail acquiring an additional one annually after the third year. When brought into the laboratory in winter in a torpid state, an electric shock had been communicated to it, which threw it into a state of extreme excitement. Two tortoises, nearly torpid, were also put by the professor into a glass bell filled with laughing gas, and they immediately began to leap about with great agility, and continued in this state of muscular excitement for more than an hour.[52]

Shepard had visited many localities throughout the United States and Canada in the course of accumulating his cabinets, and in 1839 he made the first of a number of trips to Europe. He gathered the finest specimens he could find, minerals and meteorites, fossils and shells. A younger colleague who catalogued many of the Amherst cabinets in the 1870s recounted that

> Shepard had developed a genius for collecting. As professor at the Charleston Medical School, he had all the doctors in all the mountain regions collecting for him. For more than a generation he had a monopoly of all the rich regions of the South from his winter residence there, and also collected from all the best localities in the North, discovering many of them himself, and every year going to Europe with a great store for exchange, until his mineral collection became so large that he could rarely get anything new.[53]

Gathering meteorites, Shepard was eager not only to examine specimens but also to learn about the circumstances under which they had occurred. One of his correspondents over many years was Edward C. Herrick. They exchanged celestial observations and memoranda about falling stars, fireballs, supposed meteorite observations, and places where local lore recorded falls of strange rocks or 'astrolites.' He requested any information Herrick might have of falls of meteors during the last twenty years. Shepard was particularly curious about reports from Pennsylvania of an apparent meteorite fall some sixteen years before, 'for some facts have lately come to my notice which point pretty distinctly to a certain large three still ingloriously reposing in the bosom of mother earth, into which it was thrust from out of the heavens in the presence of a reputable witness now living here!!'[54] In the *Journal* he reported and described various meteorites and fragments, and analyzed their composition. He collected communications on how meteorites had been found and on what had become of them. According to a letter about one 'meteoric mass,'

> It was found several years since by a laborer, on the plantation of Mr. Samuel M. McKeown, which is situated about six and a half miles below this place, on the Columbia road. His first impression on ploughing it up, was, that it was exceedingly heavy for its size, he took it to the house, where, however, it excited no particular attention, and was accordingly suffered to remain behind an out-building until very recently, when the finder had the curiosity to take it to the blacksmith, who at once proved it to be malleable. He cut several pieces from the mass, out of which he made horse-shoes, nails and hinges for a gate. The original weight of the mass was thirty-six pounds.[55]

Shepard then gave an account of the remainder of the mass, which had since come into his possession, its content and peculiarities of appearance, adding to a veritable catalogue of meteorites and their histories in the pages of the *American Journal of Science.*

Shepard's appointment to the faculty at Amherst brought his outstanding collections to the college. Shepard and his family were friends of Edward Hitchcock, professor of natural history at Amherst, and Hitchcock had been an assistant in Silliman's laboratory years before and a periodic visitor to New Haven since. Shepard carried minerals on some trips between New Haven and Amherst, letters on others. Through the years he was often called upon when transportation was difficult to arrange. When he went to England in 1839, he took along specimens of Connecticut Valley sandstone that Hitchcock believed showed impressions of drops of rain.[56] A letter from Hitchcock to Benjamin Silliman, Jr. asked him to 'send the package of chemicals from Mr Shepard to Hartford by the railroad & to the care of Brown & Parsons booksellers if he thinks this can be done safely.'[57] And so the round of communication within Silliman's circle continued.

When Hitchcock became president of Amherst College in 1845, the trustees 'at the same time elected Prof. Charles U. Shepard, of New Haven, professor of chemistry and natural history, "to take effect provided Professor Hitchcock accepts the presidency."'[58] Accordingly, in 1847 Shepard resigned his appointment at Yale and, upon the

completion of a fireproof building to house his collections, they came
to Amherst and the Woods cabinet.

Shepard continued to teach each winter at the Medical College in
Charleston—he had received an honorary M.D. from Dartmouth in
1836—returning to New Haven after his lectures and thence to Amherst. After 1852 his title in Amherst College was professor of natural
history,[59] but Hitchcock recorded that 'Professor Shepard, I believe, has
not lectured on any branch of natural history except mineralogy and
astrolithology.'[60] Amherst gave him the LL.D. in 1857.

The warm relationship between the Shepards and the Sillimans
continued, reflected in the letters to and from Charleston each winter.
For some years Mrs. Shepard had not been well, 'She was both from
form and temperament inclined to the consumption,'[61] and it was
hoped that the Charleston climate would benefit her health. On
arriving in that city in the fall of 1849, Mrs. Shepard's letter to Mrs.
Silliman read, 'We found the weather oppressively hot & the yellow
fever quite prevalent. . . . Mr Shepard has been the only one who has
been out during the day.' She had hoped to stay longer in New Haven
'that I might have further opportunity of seeing you,'[62] for Mrs.
Silliman was then ill. Charles Shepard wrote to Silliman of their worry
over Mrs. Silliman's health. 'It was very sad for us to view her so feeble
as we did at our parting glance; and this farewell view of one whom
Mrs S. & myself have always placed next to our own mothers in the
affection with which we regarded her, contributed to render the
departure more painful than any we have ever before experienced.'[63]

After Mrs. Silliman's death, Silliman found comfort with the
Shepards. 'Our friends the Shepards having returned from Charleston Julia & I passed the evening of this day with them at their cottage
and I read to them the account of Mrs Silliman contained in the preceding number of this journal and they were intensely interested and
gratified and my own sorrow was quickened again but soothed by sweet
consolations.'[64]

Mrs. Shepard's own health continued to fail despite three trips
abroad. 'These voyages were palliative and the winters passed in
Carolina tended also to lengthen the life of the patient,' Silliman wrote
in his 'Personal Notices' in 1854. 'Decidedly in a fixed consumption' in
May, she died on 1 October, '. . . a lovely Christian lady—decided and
consistent.'[65] The bond between Shepard and Silliman had sustained
both through personal sorrow.

Silliman's influence on his many students and assistants was one that seemed stronger as time passed and they went on to teach others. In 1851 Shepard wrote to Silliman from Charleston:

> As I look back to 20 or 25 years ago, it occurs to me as a curious reflection that four persons who were members of your class, or in your laboratory have now under their instruction by lectures, some hundreds of young men in the same or very similar branches—I refer to Dr. Hitchcock, Prof. Hubbard, your son, & myself. Thus may the useful work go on. . . .[66]

At Amherst, Shepard's magnificent collections grew larger. In 1859 the American Association for the Advancement of Science met in Springfield, and an excursion to Amherst College was conducted by Professor Hitchcock. The visitors marveled at Hitchcock's cabinet of footprints in the sandstone of the Connecticut River Valley, and at Shepard's collections. In the *Journal* an account of the meeting contained this description of Shepard's meteorites and minerals:

> Whatever the *Black stone* of Mecca may prove to be, meteorite or porphyry, the scientific pilgrim to Amherst will be rewarded by an inspection of the largest and most important collection of meteoric specimens in the world, excepting that of the Imperial Museum of Vienna. By the untiring exertions of Prof. Shepard, 124 meteoric discharges are here represented, in choice and unblemished specimens. The Vienna cabinet is stated in Mr. Haidinger's report of Jan. 7, 1859 to contain 137 localities.
>
> The mineralogical collection of Prof. Shepard at Amherst is worthy of most particular notice. In the richness and splendor of its selections, the mineral species are nowhere in America and seldom anywhere so well represented. Choice specimens seem to have come to this celebrated collector's hands like the fabled fish of the weird fisherman. Whatever was most rare or choice from any locality appears to have found no rest until it was safely placed on his shelves.[67]

The letters from Charleston meanwhile reflected the changes there as Shepard wrote in 1859 to Silliman:

> The lectures have been well attended considering that they commenced during the prevalence of yellow fever. . . . Alas! time disease & misfortune have made sad changes among many families who were high in prosperity when I first came to Charleston. It seems to me that these mournful inroads and subversions have been more palpable here than elsewhere. The shuttle seems to fly faster in the loom of human life within the tropics than in the temperate zone.[68]

At the end of 1860 he discussed the feeling of separateness in the South in a long letter. 'Very few go to the North now for education.

Northern teachers & even clergymen are becoming almost unknown.'
And he worried about the future and the position of the southern states.
He foresaw an explosion 'into scores of asteroids, comets and meteorites. . . .'[69] But he remained in his beloved Charleston until 1861 and
was recalled in 1865 to resume his teaching at the Medical College 'at
the urgent invitation of his former colleagues.'[70] In the meantime he
had traveled again to Europe and, with a commission to purchase
specimens for Amherst, 'early stumbled upon some very good collections of fossils'; Professor Hitchcock especially requested that he check
on the casts of the Megatherium to find if they had been sent to the
college, for, Hitchcock wrote, 'We hear nothing of it yet.'[71]

In 1869 Shepard resigned his professorship at Charleston, and was
succeeded by his son, but continued to lecture there for many years
afterward.[72] At Amherst he held his chair until 1877, but spent more
time with his collections, teaching for a shorter part of the year. The
young professor who began teaching at Amherst in 1870, and who
ordered the cabinets for Shepard's collections, gave his impressions of
Shepard, his 'exquisite politeness' and his 'genial lawlessness.'[73]

> Gradually his life all centered in his collections, and he appeared annually
> in Amherst only for the short spring term, and with a genial and
> apparently unconscious disregard for the rules and regulations applying
> to professors in general would send a very polite note to the President
> saying that he would meet the senior class at twelve o'clock during the rest
> of the year. He then fastened a row of chairs on the long lecture room table
> for a back row of seniors, the middle row sitting on the table, and the front
> row in chairs on the floor. The professor could then hold his beautiful
> crystals before the nose of each man. If a student attempted to touch a
> specimen, he drew back and guarded his precious crystal with a gesture of
> the most affectionate solicitude. He was always interesting, drawing easily
> from a great fund of knowledge and experience, and speaking with courtly
> dignity and faultless English.[74]

The conditions under which the college might eventually purchase the Shepard collections had been agreed upon when he came to
Amherst: when he reached seventy the college might buy them for two-
thirds of their value, but for no more than $40,000. Though their worth
far exceeded this, they were bought for the sum named.[75] They had, of
course, been deposited in the college buildings all along. Then, one
night during spring recess in 1882, fire destroyed Walker Hall, the
building now housing the collections. Benjamin Emerson, the young
professor who had by then catalogued thousands of specimens in the
cabinets, remembered how the fire broke out: '. . . from spontaneous

combustion of the floor dressing. . . . When I came in sight of the building it was a mass of flames, and of a sudden it was all tinted green and I said, "there go my datholites (a boric acid mineral which tints the flame green)."'[76] Most of Shepard's collections were destroyed—tourmalines from Paris, Maine were rescued through a window. But Shepard determined to build up another collection, and this was later given by his son, Prof. Charles Upham Shepard, Jr. of Charleston, to Amherst.[77]

Though among his contributions to mineralogy Shepard named a number of minerals, discovering several that were new, and though he wrote a number of papers on geological subjects as well, Benjamin Silliman, Jr. considered Shepard's discovery of phosphate deposits in South Carolina his greatest contribution, remarking in 1874:

> No observation or original research of Dr. Shepard has been fruitful of so much good in its consequences as his discovery, about 25 years ago, of the deposit of phosphate of lime in the Eocene marl of South Carolina, and the distinct recognition of the fact of its great value for agriculture. This discovery led, in 1859-60, to finding, in the immediate vicinity of Charleston, the richest phosphates directly above and upon the Eocene, and to its introduction into commerce on a vast scale, and the manufacture of superphosphate fertilizers, not alone for this country, but for foreign export, and the growth in consequence of an important industry in the chemical arts at Charleston.[78]

By extending the practical applications and benefits of science in his discovery of phosphates, Shepard realized one of Benjamin Silliman's aims for science. Shepard was a member of learned societies in his own country and abroad, including the Society of Natural Science of Vienna, the Imperial Society of Naturalists of St. Petersburg, and the Royal Society of Göttingen.[79]

His manners and methods as a teacher were storied at Amherst:

> Through long residence in Europe he had acquired the perfect manner of a cultivated Frenchman,—he would have said of the cultivated Englishman. It was the habit of the rude sophomore to bow to him on the street. He would remove his hat and make a most courtly bow to the retreating form of the crude native.
>
> His audience was small but interested. Sometimes he called the roll for a little while, and when one man directly in front of him answered for half a dozen, he pointed to him with an expression of deepest interest and asked, 'What *is* your name?'[80]

He made 'organic chemistry a thing of beauty' at Charleston, and it was recalled at the Medical College that 'no teacher was ever more beloved and respected by such a heterogeneous body of pupils.'[81]

In Shepard's career as scientist and teacher, Silliman had been both guide and friend, for, as Shepard remarked in a tribute to Silliman: 'Though he loved knowledge of every kind, and delighted in its communication, he valued goodness most of all. The highest excellence of his character consisted of his desire to advance others.'[82] Silliman's influence thus reached throughout his circle and then spread far beyond. The Charleston memoriam of Shepard on 2 May 1886 read: 'He doubtless was fired by the gigantic strides which natural science had taken in the early part of the nineteenth century, and the seed sown by the scientists of that time did not fall upon barren ground.'[83]

NOTES

[1] Silliman, 'Reminiscences,' V, 89, Silliman Family Papers.

[2] Shepard to George P. Fisher, 10 August 1865, in Fisher, *Silliman*, II, 371.

[3] Silliman, 'Personal Notcies,' XVI, 6 (8 October 1855, 'Tour to Amherst,') Silliman Family Papers.

[4] Silliman, 'Reminiscences,' V, 65.

[5] *News and Courier* (Charleston), 2 May 1886.

[6] Shepard to Fisher, in Fisher, *Silliman*, II, 370.

[7] Tyler, *History of Amherst College During its First Half Century*, p. 622.

[8] Hitchcock, *Reminiscences*, p. 101; Amherst College, *Biographical Record*, p. 17.

[9] Tyler, *History of Amherst College During its First Half Century*, pp. 622-623.

[10] Hitchcock, *Reminiscences*, p. 101.

[11] Amherst College, *Biographical Record*, p. 17.

[12] Shepard to Fisher, in Fisher, *Silliman*, II, 370.

[13] Silliman, 'Reminiscences,' V, 61.

[14] Charles U. Shepard, 'Address of Presentation,' in *Memorial Addresses*, pp. 9-10.

[15] Silliman, 'Personal Notices,' XIV, 270, 1 October 1854, Silliman Family Papers.

[16] *Ibid.*, XIV, 272.

[17] George C. Shepard to Charles Upham Shepard, 1 March 1830, Shepard Papers, Amherst.

[18] George C. Shepard to Charles Upham Shepard, 4 May 1830, Shepard Papers, Amherst.

[19] Silliman, 'Reminiscences,' V, 62. Silliman Family Papers. The appointment was probably made in 1830, for the title appears in article headings in the *American Journal of Science* in 1830.

[20] *Ibid.*, V, 62.

[21] *Ibid.*, V, 63.

[22] Shepard, *Franklin Institution.*

[23] Silliman, 'Reminiscences,' V, 63, Silliman Family Papers.

[24] *Ibid.*, V, 64.

[25] *Ibid.*, VI, 162.

[26] Memorandum in Shepard Papers, Amherst.

[27] Letter of Silliman, Shepard Papers, Amherst.

[28] Silliman to Shepard, 25 December 1832, Shepard Papers, Amherst.

[29] Silliman, 'Reminiscences,' VI, 63, Silliman Family Papers.

[30] Review of Charles Upham Shepard, *Treatise on Mineralogy*, in *Am. J. Sci.*, 1832, *22*, 395.

[31] Shepard, *Treatise on Mineralogy*, I, iii.

[32] Silliman, 'Reminiscences,' V, 62, Silliman Family Papers.

[33] 'Mr. C. U. Shepard's private school of Mineralogy and other Branches of Natural History,' *Am. J. Sci.*, 1834, *26*, 215.

[34] Charles Upham Shepard, 'Datholite and Iolite in Connecticut,' *Am. J. Sci.*, 1832, *22*, 389.

[35] Gilman, *Dana*, p. 32; Silliman, 'Reminiscences,' V, 78, Silliman Family Papers.

[36] Gilman, *Dana*, p. 37.

[37] Silliman, 'Reminiscences,' V, 78, Silliman Family Papers.

[38] *Ibid.*, V, 65.

[39] *News and Courier* (Charleston), 2 May 1886.

[40] 'Geological Survey of Connecticut,' *Am. J. Sci.*, 1835, *28*, 381.

[41] Percival, *Geology of the State of Connecticut*, [p. 2].

[42] Shepard, *Geological Survey of Connecticut.*

[43] South Carolina, Medical College, Charleston. *Annual Announcement* 1837–1838.

[44] *Ibid.*

[45] Silliman to Shepard, 22 February 1838, Shepard Papers, Amherst.

[46] *Ibid.*, 9 September 1838.

[47] Shepard to Silliman, 3 January 1843, De Forest Family Papers.

[48] Silliman, 'Personal Notices,' X, 2 February 1845, ff., Silliman Family Papers.

[49] *Ibid.*, X, 4 February 1845.

[50] D. A. Dobson to F. B. Higgins, 28 January 1845, Higgins Papers.

[51] Letter (n. d.) of Middleton Michel, '46, professor of physiology from 1869–94,

quoted in Waring, *History of Medicine in South Carolina* p. 82. Original in possession of Mrs. Heard Robertson, Augusta, Georgia.

[52] Lyell, *Second Visit to the United States*, I, 229.

[53] Benjamin K. Emerson, 'The Geological and Mineralogical Collections of Amherst College,' *Amherst Graduates' Quart.*, 1915-16, 5, 22-23.

[54] Shepard to Herrick, 10 September 1839, Herrick Papers.

[55] Charles Upham Shepard, 'On Meteoric Iron in South Carolina,' *Am. J. Sci.*, 1849, *2nd ser. 7*, 449.

[56] Hitchcock to Silliman, 22 July 1839, Hitchcock Papers.

[57] Hitchcock to Silliman, Jr., 20 August 1840, Hitchcock Papers.

[58] Tyler, *History of Amherst College . . . From 1821 to 1891*, p. 106.

[59] Amherst College, *Biographical Record*, p. 17.

[60] Hitchcock, *Reminiscences*, p. 291.

[61] Silliman, 'Personal Notices,' XIV, 270, Silliman Family Papers.

[62] Harriet Taylor Shepard to Mrs. Silliman, 20 November 1849, Silliman Family Papers.

[63] Shepard to Silliman, 21 November 1849, Silliman Family Papers.

[64] Silliman, 'Personal Notices,' XIV, 44, Silliman Family Papers.

[65] *Ibid.*, XIV, 271.

[66] Shepard to Silliman, 21 December 1851, De Forest Family Papers.

[67] 'The Thirteenth Meeting of the American Association for the Advancement of Science,' *Am. J. Sci.*, 1859, *2nd ser. 28*, 293.

[68] Shepard to Silliman, 13 February 1859, De Forest Family Papers.

[69] *Ibid.*, 30 December 1860.

[70] *News and Courier* (Charleston), 2 May 1886.

[71] Hitchcock to Shepard, 4 August 1863, De Forest Family Papers.

[72] 'Minutes of the Faculty of the Medical College of the State of South Carolina,' 27 February and 8 March 1869; *News and Courier* (Charleston), 2 May 1866.

[73] Emerson (n. 53), p. 22.

[74] *Ibid.*, p. 23.

[75] *Ibid.*, p. 22.

[76] *Ibid.*, p. 97.

[77] *Ibid.*, p. 98. Harriet Silliman Shepard, married to John William De Forest, predeceased her father; Shepard's daughter Fanny was married to Charles Pinckney James, a professor of law who was Justice of the Supreme Court of the District of Columbia. De Forest Family Papers.

[78] Silliman [Jr.], *American Contributions to Chemistry*, p. 75.

[79] *News and Courier* (Charleston), 2 May 1886; 'Obituary, Charles Upham Shepard, *Am. J. Sci.*, 1886, *3rd ser. 31*, 483.

[80] Emerson (n. 53), p. 23.

[81] Robert Wilson, 'Their Shadowy Influence Still Hovers About Medical College,' *News and Courier* (Charleston), 13 April 1913.

[82] Shepard (n. 14), p. 12.

[83] *News and Courier* (Charleston), 2 May 1886.

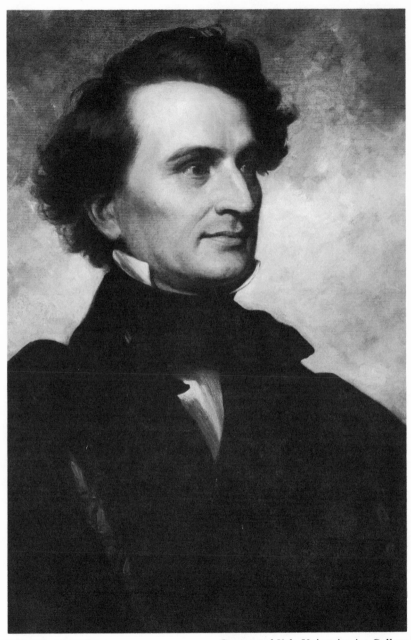

James Dwight Dana, by Daniel Huntington.

A Portrait of James Dwight Dana

MARGARET W. ROSSITER

JAMES DWIGHT DANA was in many ways Benjamin Silliman's greatest student and one of the most prominent American scientists of the nineteenth century. In addition Dana's personal ties to Professor Silliman were especially close, since he married Silliman's daughter, moved in with the family, and succeeded Silliman at the *Journal* and on the Yale faculty. As such Dana was the heir of all that Silliman had done for science at Yale.

As a young man Dana traveled extensively—east to Smyrna in Turkey and west to Australia, the Philippines and around the world— but he always returned to Yale and to the tradition in natural history and conservative religion that Benjamin Silliman had established there. In the 1850s, after his marriage to Silliman's daughter Henrietta and amidst the constant comings and goings of both Sillimans, Dana emerged as the mainstay of the family's scientific interests in New Haven. He not only managed and edited the *American Journal of Science*, lectured on geology and mineralogy, raised funds for the Yale Scientific School, and upheld the harmony of science and religion, but he also wrote such major works in mineralogy, geology, and invertebrate zoology that at an early age he became widely known as one of the nation's most outstanding scientists. Dana's achievements certainly warmed Professor Silliman's heart, but Dana's nervous breakdown and relapses after 1859 also distressed 'Uncle Ben' greatly. Dana was not as hardy as the Sillimans, but his long and productive career, which lasted into the 1890s, contributed greatly to the growth and reputation of American science.

Although many of his fellow American scientists have been characterized as Baconian 'fact-gatherers,'[1] Dana showed at an early age that he had a much broader and more idealistic philosophical orientation than such a description would allow. Between 1838 and

Any biographer of James Dwight Dana faces the problem that though the man and his wife both maintained large correspondences, disappointingly few letters are to or from the Sillimans, with whom they interacted most strongly. Only when someone was away from Hillhouse Avenue was there need to write a letter. Such letters, as those to Benjamin Silliman, Jr. when he was in Louisville, are infrequent but among the most informative about Dana's true feelings. Also very useful are Dana's letters to George Brush in Europe in the 1850s and his wife's to Harriet Trumbull in 1859-60. Unfortunately Dana seems not to have kept a diary.

1842 Dana had the extreme good fortune to travel to the South Seas with the Wilkes Expedition and thereby gain, as had Charles Darwin on the *Beagle* a few years before, an awareness and familiarity with far larger problems of geological change than he ever could have acquired at home in New Haven. The ambivalent way in which Dana faced these larger questions reveals, however, a certain underlying tension or inconsistency in his thought. On the one hand, he had a very open, direct, and flexible personality. His work in mineralogy showed that in the early 1850s, when European schools were arguing over changes in classification, Dana was able to mediate between the warring factions and make the necessary changes in long-held doctrine. Despite this open and direct Dana, whose theories dispassionately reflected the latest discoveries regardless of the consequences, there was another side to his character. He also held a strong and relatively inflexible personal religious faith which persisted in seeing a Divine Plan in all of nature, even after the *Origin of Species* had presented an alternative to such an ordered and purposive world view. Rather than confront such a challenge immediately, Dana, already under psychological pressure from other quarters, suffered a nervous and physical breakdown in 1859 and could not read the *Origin of Species* for several years. For a long time he seemed to lack the mental strength to face the whole issue, and it is only through occasional hints in the 1870s and 1880s that we can understand how he did grapple with evolution in later years.

Likewise Dana's temperament was exemplary up to a point, but then revealed certain serious limitations. On the surface he seems to have been a quiet individual, who with strong discipline and determination went briskly about his daily tasks in New Haven. In such a serene and harmonious setting, surrounded by like-thinking colleagues and family, Dana was able to accomplish gargantuan tasks at a rapid pace and seemed utterly stable, the model of judicious restraint, even when provoked by his colleagues' professional squabbles. But Dana was also a delicate and high-strung individual, and when he suffered a personal loss, felt that his strongly-held religious and philosophical views were under attack, or felt threatened or in conflict in any way, he quickly lost his usual control and forbearance and lashed out strongly at his critic. At other times, even that was too much for him and he collapsed under the strain. Unfortunately we have no diaries or autobiography and few letters which would reveal more of this deeper, more private, and vulnerable Dana. The image he presented to the public, however, the Dana we might have met at the AAAS, written to about the *Journal*, or met on Hillhouse Avenue in New Haven, was in full control of his emotions and is plentifully documented. To him we now turn.

James Dwight Dana was born in Utica, New York on 12 February 1813, the son of a country merchant and the eldest of ten children. He seems to have had a happy boyhood around the family store and an aunt recalled him later as a 'merry boy, always ready for game of romps.' He also enjoyed collecting natural history specimens and had an extensive 'cabinet' even before the age of ten.[2] He attended local schools and in 1827 entered Utica High School, whose curriculum was based on that of the famed Round Hill School in Massachusetts and featured field trips and natural history. In 1829 Asa Gray came to teach at the school and, though it is not known whether he taught Dana, the two became acquainted about this time and were in correspondence by 1833.[3] Despite the large size of his family, Mr. Dana was able to send his bright son off to college. Young James chose Yale, attracted, as he later recalled, by the fame of Professor Silliman, then about fifty, and the Gibbs mineral collection.[4] Though Dana did not yet expect to pursue a career in science, he planned to study natural history and geology while preparing to enter a profession.

At Yale, where Dana enrolled as a sophomore in October 1830, he took the standard curriculum of classics and science, excelling in mathematics, botany, and mineralogy. Although little is known of his activities at college, Professor Silliman would later recommend him as showing 'ingenuity, industry and perseverance,'[5] a characterization that would describe his whole life quite aptly. Dana's closest friend was Edward C. Herrick, the son of a local minister, who worked in a nearby bookstore and who shared Dana's strong interest in natural history.[6] At Yale, Dana also learned a great deal of mineralogy from Charles U. Shepard who was teaching the subject there in the 1830s. In his almost three years at Yale, Dana came to love the scientific atmosphere of New Haven. For him it had already become a warm intellectual home, where he had friends who shared his scientific interests and with whom he could discuss natural history far into the night.

Upon completion of his studies at Yale, Dana did not take up medicine, as might have been expected, since he found it 'disgusting.' Instead he postponed his career decision for a year. Indulging a desire for adventure, in August 1833 he sailed for the Mediterranean as a mathematics instructor on the government ship *Delaware*. His parents' fears concerning such a long journey must have been partially allayed by their knowledge that should he meet with difficulty he could call upon an uncle who was a missionary in Constantinople. Although Dana's original aim had been to visit Paris and perhaps study there, nothing came of this plan. Nevertheless he put this unusual year abroad to excellent use, and it in turn determined his commitment to become a scientist. When on board ship, he studied conchology and crystallography; when on land he collected shells, plants, and minerals, and purchased scientific books. Whenever and wherever possible, he also observed meteors and geological phenomena, such as Mt. Vesuvius, which he described in a letter to Professor Silliman, later published in the *Journal*. Dana also used every opportunity to try to find a Hessian fly in Europe. Before he left, he and Herrick had been studying this agricultural pest, about which little was known, and Dana wished to prove that it was not a strictly American insect. Great was his excitement when he found one in Italy in April 1834 and could report his success to Herrick.[7] In general, Dana took far more delight in his scientific exploits abroad than in the exotic cultures he was visiting, for he found the cities of the Middle East 'filthy' and the inhabitants 'rascals' who were full of cheating and trickery.

Although his interests in this year abroad ranged over all of natural history, Dana also began to focus his studies more specifically on mineralogy and crystallography. Whether he had studied crystallography with Shepard is unclear, but his recalculation, on board ship, of the angles and dimensions of the crystals in William Phillips' *Elementary Introduction to Mineralogy* (1823) was an impressive feat.[8] At this time Dana also devised some improvements in H. J. Brooke's crystallographic symbols, which he published with Shepard's warm encouragement upon his return to New Haven.[9] During the voyage Dana also read a classic article by Berzelius on the chemical arrangement of minerals. Characteristically he plunged into this unorthodox system, ambitiously made some 'improvements,' and sent them off to Berzelius, who responded with some criticisms a year later.[10] Shepard was sufficiently impressed with Dana's new system that he published it as an appendix to Part II of his own *Treatise on Mineralogy* in 1835. Dana's capacity for hard work and independent thought as well as his aptitude for mineralogy were already quite evident by the time he returned to New Haven in December 1834. They would become even more evident in the years ahead.

Shortly after Dana's return to the United States, Benjamin Silliman offered him a position as assistant in his geological lectures at Yale, a job which required Dana to lay out the rock specimens for the lecture and which consumed only three hours per day. This position was something of a prize for it was one of the few such assistantships available at a major research center at the time, and over the years it had had a distinguished roster of appointees. Winning the job was fortunate for Dana, since he could now report to his father that he was employed, but, he wrote Silliman, he would have stayed on in New Haven even if the post had not been offered. Of all the places he might go, 'there is no other in our Country equally pleasant for study.' The New Haven facilities, he wrote his father, were such that if he remained there he could 'ride with the current' rather than be left to himself as he would in Utica.[11] He had, in effect, ambitiously decided on a scientific career and for the next few years would need all the resources New Haven had to offer.

Dana remained in New Haven for three years working feverishly on natural history, especially mineralogy. He and Edward Herrick became the chief participants in the Yale Natural History Society which, during its brief existence, provided the support and criticism a departmental seminar might today. Almost all of Dana's papers in the 1830s were initially read to the society. His major project at this time was the writing of a complete *System of Mineralogy*. Although Charles Shepard was then publishing Part II of his own text, a compilation of all known minerals listed alphabetically with their characteristics, Dana followed in the European tradition and made the more ambitious attempt to arrange the minerals in an order revealing their similarities or 'natural affinities.' His system, completed in May 1837, was based largely on that of the German mineralogist Friedrich Mohs, the successor of Abraham Werner at the Freiberg School of Mines and the dominant influence in mineralogy at the time. Like Mohs, Dana frequently used analogies among the three natural kingdoms of zoology, botany, and mineralogy to explain phenomena, a style of reasoning he would use throughout his life, sometimes to his detriment. The most notable characteristic of Dana's 570-page compendium was its coverage of the diverse and extensive literature on mineralogy that Dana had read and mastered in Professor Silliman's library. The *System* was an impressive volume from a man only twenty-four years old and far surpassed Shepard's modest effort. Dana moved promptly to the forefront of American mineralogists and aroused great hopes among his countrymen.

Dana's work in mineralogy in the 1830s also demonstrated that he was more than an industrious compiler. His approach was to start with the problem of classification, question the theory behind the prevailing system, ponder its scientific and philosophical basis, and then come to a broad theoretical grasp of the processes involved. In his *System* of 1837 and more extensively in an 1836 article on twin crystals,[12] Dana questioned how minerals were formed, a basic problem in geochemistry. He accepted William Hyde Wollaston's idea that atoms were like spheres but rejected the notion that they were held together by 'cohesion.' He argued instead that such a force should act equally strongly in all directions, but some minerals, especially the twin crystals, showed that it did not. Dana preferred the idea that the atoms in minerals arranged themselves according to the degree of 'attractive force' which they felt for the three electrical axes. Thus the reason a crystal might be elongated in one direction would be that one axis was stronger than the others. Dana's views were apparently original and correct, although similar views based on polarizing forces were already popular among the adherents of Naturphilosophie in Germany. This whole subject of 'crystallogeny' was an active area of research in mineralogy between 1835 and 1855 and would again attract Dana's attention later on.

Absorbed as he was, Dana felt in the mid-1830s that he should not leave New Haven until he was better prepared for a scientific career; he resisted job offers from Dartmouth and Middlebury colleges. Then in August 1836, while he was still busy with his *System*, he heard of a very different opportunity: the formation of the United States Exploring Expedition to the South Seas, to be gone several years in pursuit of scientific data. Although Dana had vowed after his last voyage never again to have anything to do with the navy, his friend Asa Gray persuaded him to apply for the post of geologist/mineralogist to the expedition at a handsome annual salary of $2,500. Dana became eager to make the trip and urged his friend Herrick to do likewise, for it promised to open whole new worlds to them.

Unfortunately there were numerous delays before the expedition left Norfolk, Virginia in August 1838. In the interim Dana underwent an important religious conversion at New Haven in April and May 1838. Although his family was devoutly Christian and he had made it a point to attend Sunday services in New Haven, Dana had not felt strongly religious. Now, however, on the eve of his anticipated departure for a lengthy and dangerous voyage and influenced by his family's accounts of a religious revival in Utica, Dana felt called to deepen his commitment to God. Although little is known of his conversion, his religious feelings were to become much more noticeable in his scientific work and correspondence. His religious views quickly fused with his already idealistic philosophical orientation, and he became anxious to see a 'Divine Plan' as well as 'force' and 'unity' everywhere in nature. In particular, he wished to reserve a role for God in both geological change and the creation of species. Later Dana was also influenced by Professor Silliman's concern for defending the harmony of science and religion; and when the issue grew more virulent in the 1850s, Dana, to Silliman's delight, took an active role in the controversy.

On the Wilkes Expedition, Dana, as one of the seven scientists on board, was officially in charge of geology and mineralogy. Later changes in personnel gave him zoophytes and crustaceans as well. The squadron's first major stop was in Rio de Janeiro, where the crew spent six weeks refitting the ships and touring the area. They then had a harrowing voyage around Cape Horn with a gale that lasted three days and three nights and wrecked two of the packet ships. Judging from Dana's dramatic accounts of the stormy passage, it must have given religion to those who did not have it already. Arriving in Valparaiso, Chile in April 1839, Dana and the other 'scientifics' took advantage of their time on land to investigate the Cordilleras. After a stop in Callao, Peru they left South America for the exotic islands of Tahiti, popularly known to Americans as the site of a Christian mission and a stop for whaling ships. Dana spent three weeks investigating the coral reefs before the expedition pushed on to Samoa and then to Sydney. From December 1839 to February 1840, while Captain Wilkes explored parts of Antarctica, Dana and the rest of the scientific corps studied the Australian coastline and sailed on to New Zealand. Rejoining Wilkes, the whole crew sailed north to the Tonga Islands and the Fijis, where they arrived in August 1840 and spent three months. Unfortunately the tribes on Fiji were so hostile, even cannibalistic, that they not only curtailed Dana's coral investigations but also murdered two of the crewmen! After this unhappy episode, Dana's ship, the *Peacock*, headed for Hawaii (via Samoa) and the Columbia River in the northwestern United States, but as it attempted to land, the ship caught on the shoals and was wrecked by the breakers. Fortunately all survived, although the collections on board (only a part of the total) were lost. Again Dana must have felt that God was protecting him from the catastrophes that befell the group. Back on land, the weary crew headed for San Francisco. There they purchased a new ship, the *Oregon*, and prepared to return to the east coast. Although the expedition had already been at sea for three years, Captain Wilkes nevertheless decided to return the long way around. They set sail in July 1841 and, after stops at Manila, Singapore, and Capetown, arrived in New York in June 1842. The whole crew was glad to be back. Dana's family and friends were thankful for his safe return and anxious to hear more about his adventures.[13]

Upon their return to the United States, Dana and the other scientists faced the task of arranging and reporting on their vast collections. Dana's job was immense. His three fields would require several years' work, and, although others would not complete all their volumes for various reasons, Dana stuck doggedly to his task and finished his third volume ten years later. The next twelve years, 1843–54, were in fact the most productive of Dana's long life. Besides three expedition reports, he also put out three new editions of his *System of Mineralogy* and wrote a mineralogical textbook. Supported by a government salary of $1,440 (compared to the $1,200 salary for Yale faculty at the time), Dana devoted himself exclusively to his work. He put in six hours a day, took few vacations, declined the various lecture tours and consulting jobs that occupied and sidetracked so many of his contemporaries, and alternated his work between the mineralogy and the expedition reports. It seemed almost as if, rather than take a vacation, he did one as relaxation from the other! If two portraits in Gilman's biography are any indication, he thrived on such a regimen, for Dana hardly changed in physical appearance between his portraits of 1843 and 1857. In both, with his intense eyes, sharp nose, and untamed curly brown hair, he looks erect, vigorous, and youthful.

Dana's work from 1843 to 1854 shows his increasing maturity, incessant activity, growing concern with issues of unity and development, and, in geology, his mounting confidence, almost to the point of arrogance, in a theistic world view. His impact on the various fields to which he contributed varied widely. In mineralogy the fourth edition of Dana's *System* (1854) resolved a century-long controversy. Subsequent editions remain to this day the established authority in the field. In geology, Dana's work, though sober, fair, and important in particulars, was representative of a particular viewpoint rather than decisive on major issues. In marine zoology he contributed to two areas. He did a masterly study of the zoophytes or corals (Anthora, Actinoida, and a few Hydroida) which was the first thorough study of that group and today stands relatively unchallenged. With Crustacea, the field, he wrote William Redfield in 1839, that he liked least of his assignments, his work was useful but unexciting and has since been discredited. To all three fields, however, his contributions were momentous, for even when his conclusions were in error, his observations proved useful to others.

During the first three years after the expedition, 1843 to 1846, Dana, first in Washington and then in New Haven, revised his *System of Mineralogy* and completed his volume on zoophytes. Both were tedious, time-consuming tasks. Dana was anxious to revise the mineralogy book to include the numerous new species and localities that workers on the state geological surveys had discovered since 1837. Although he was eager to include all new species, both foreign and domestic, he especially wanted his book to stand as the authority on American minerals. For this he again exhausted Professor Silliman's library and whatever books he could find in Washington. Although he had considerable trouble finding a publisher for the book, once out it received favorable notice from at least two of the leading mineralogists of Europe, Wilhelm Haidinger, Mohs' successor in Vienna, and Carl Rammelsberg of Berlin.[14]

When Dana turned in 1844 from mineralogy to his work on marine biology for the Wilkes Expedition, he found the classification of zoophytes beset with difficulties. Not only was it a miscellany of creatures that had little in common, it was also the least studied area in the animal kingdom. Although Lamarck, Blainville, Ehrenberg, and Milne-Edwards had worked with some of the species and a few were contained in collections in Boston and Philadelphia, Dana found that most of these had been imperfectly described and classified. This chaotic state was not surprising since the zoophytes were particularly difficult to work with, they reproduced by asexual budding and so lacked even rudimentary sexual organs. Dana finally decided to use the nervous system as the basis for his classification, and his volume on zoophytes, which appeared with an atlas in 1846, contained descriptions of 267 species of which 203 were new. Dana and the Wilkes Expedition had certainly given a needed boost to the new science of marine zoology.

Unfortunately Dana's success with this unusual group of invertebrates emboldened him to speculate on the general principles of organic development, which he felt held true not only for a peculiar group like the zoophytes but for all the other branches of the plant and animal kingdoms as well. He formulated a 'law' that a species required only 'the concentration of a specific [minimum] amount of vital force, and a certain tributary space where this force exists' in order to reproduce itself. Although he did not go quite so far as to identify a species with a center of force, he clearly thought he had discovered one of the higher laws of nature. He admitted that his concept of force was based on an analogy with the role of chemical forces in mineral formation in inorganic nature and defended its use in a lengthy footnote. Dana showed the effects of his work in mineralogy and Naturphilosophie by finding unifying forces in the most unexpected quarters. It is perhaps worth noting that, although the book was concerned with species and their development, Dana did not make any references to the recent appearance of the *Vestiges of Creation.* The *Vestiges* had aroused considerable controversy elsewhere but left Dana surprisingly unconcerned.[15]

The period 1843 to 1846 was also an important one for Dana's personal life. He must have known Henrietta Silliman, the professor's third daughter, during his student days over a decade before, since the professor was accustomed to entertain his students in his home. But she was ten years younger than he, and the romance had not blossomed until Dana's return from the South Seas. Perhaps his exciting and heroic letters from the expedition, which had been read and reread on Hillhouse Avenue, had stirred her interest in the romantic young man. In any case they were engaged a few months after his return and were married in June 1844. At first he and Hettie lived with the Sillimans, but later they built their own house, a spacious Italianate villa, a few doors away at what is now 24 Hillhouse Avenue. Although their future was somewhat uncertain, they knew they could live on Dana's government salary for a few more years before having to seek a professorship elsewhere. In fact the possibility of leaving New Haven arose only once—in 1848 with an offer from Harvard—but wealthy friends of Professor Silliman quickly countered by endowing the new Silliman Professorship of Natural History for Dana to occupy whenever he chose. Dana thus came into the seemingly fortunate position that family and science would henceforth be so closely intertwined in his life that he could devote himself wholly to his work, assured of an understanding wife and stimulating colleagues. As it turned out this degree of 'concentration of force' was too much for Dana, and he would lean heavily on the capable Henrietta in the difficult days ahead.[16]

In 1846 Dana began his next round of activity, which centered on his *Manual of Mineralogy* (1848) for students and his volume on geology for the Wilkes Expedition (1849). In 1846 he also became an associate editor of the *American Journal of Science* and prepared several important articles for it. The Danas had their first two children, a daughter Frances and a son Edward Salisbury, who later became a mineralogist and a third generation editor of the *American Journal of Science.* The ambitious young man was settling down at home and achieving his first successes professionally.

When he discovered how outdated current textbooks on mineralogy, mostly English reprints, were, Dana decided to write one of his own. Although the market for such texts remained small and Dana's book did not sell well, he used the opportunity of writing the book to review the field critically and to take up once again the difficulties in crystallogeny or mineral formation. In an article in the *Journal,* 'On certain laws of cohesive attraction,' Dana again pointed out that the chemical force of cohesion could not account for the observed forms of minerals and went on to speculate on the nature of molecules.[17] He concluded by agreeing with Boscovitch, Faraday, and his Yale friend James D. Whelpley, who had recently written a paper on the nature of atoms,[18] that molecules were only centers of force. He hoped that if chemists would pursue this hypothesis systematically, perhaps the facts of crystallography would be explained adequately and the unity of nature restored.

Dana also turned in the mid-1840s to his second volume for the Wilkes Expedition—his massive *Geology.* In his first chapter Dana noted that 'the geology of the Pacific embraces topics of the widest importance.' In particular, he considered the topics of coral reefs, their formation and subsidence, volcanoes, ocean levels, and island location. His work on coral reefs was influenced greatly by the recent work of Charles Darwin. While in Sydney, Australia in 1839 Dana chanced on a newspaper article which described Darwin's explanation for the origin of coral atolls and barrier reefs. Dana, who had been puzzling over the problem for several months, was immediately impressed with Darwin's explanation, which, he wrote, 'threw a flood of light over the subject, and called forth feelings of peculiar satisfaction, and of gratefulness to Mr. Darwin.' During his visit to the Fijis a few months later, Dana was able to consider Darwin's theory at first hand. His own observations confirmed Darwin's theory far more completely than Darwin had thought possible.[19]

On the subject of volcanic action, Dana's examination of Mauna Loa in Hawaii and other volcanoes convinced him of the correctness of Charles Lyell's theory that lava was ejected from the top of the volcanic cone. He saw the error of Leopold von Buch, who held that the cones were built up from ejections at the bottom of horizontal sheets of lava that were elevated later.

Dana's confirmations of some of the early theories of Darwin and Lyell raise the question of Dana's relationship to the two scientists. It is a complex one for, although Dana confirmed several of each man's theories, he did not adopt all of them and became neither a uniformitarian in geology nor, in biology, an advocate of evolution until the 1880s. Several factors seemed to hold him back.

While a student at Yale, Dana may have heard of Lyell's *Principles of Geology*. Professor Silliman knew of it in 1830, discussed it with Edward Hitchcock thereafter, and may have mentioned it in his lectures.[20] Dana may also have read the *Principles* between 1834 and 1838 when he was using Professor Silliman's library for his work on mineralogy. But if not, Dana certainly read the book while on the Wilkes Expedition, for in a letter to William Redfield in June 1839, he thanked Redfield for a new edition (the fifth) of Lyell and said he found it particularly interesting for the references it made to Darwin's still unpublished *Beagle* observations. Nevertheless Lyell's work seems to have had only minor impact on Dana's thinking, and Dana hardly mentioned Lyell in the *Geology* or in a series of five articles in the *American Journal of Science* in 1846 and 1847.[21] Instead Dana used his own observations about the location of islands, coastlines, and volcanoes along certain major axes to argue for what might be termed a 'modified catastrophist' position. In brief he theorized that originally the earth had been a molten mass which had cooled, creating continental crusts in some places. He then argued, by analogy with the cooling of liquid glass into 'Prince Rupert's drops,' that the remaining fluid parts of the globe would become depressed, although in some places volcanoes would erupt to emit heat, and fissures would develop into strings of islands. The continuing contractions of the earth would be accompanied by earthquakes which would fold up mountains along the coasts of continents by horizontal compressions. Dana did not claim that his theory was original, for it agreed largely with the current views of the French geologists, Louis Élie de Beaumont and Constant Prévost, and with those of Sir Henry De la Beche, director of the Geological Survey of Great Britain. Dana's theory was in disagreement with that of von Buch.

In clinging to his catastrophist position, Dana showed both the strength of conservative religion in America, especially in the colleges and among the Silliman-Hitchcock school, and his own natural theological viewpoint. As two scholars, Philip Lawrence and Stanley Guralnick, have recently shown, Hitchcock and Silliman had, as a result of Lyell's work, slowly retreated in the late 1830s from a belief in the actual occurrence of the Mosaic Flood to a catastrophist view of the rate of geological change, which they saw as variable; they emphasized the magnitude and frequency of volcanoes, earthquakes, and later glaciers during the geological past.[22] Their continued influence diminished and distorted Lyell's uniformitarianism and its impact on Dana, and perhaps on American geologists in general. Dana could thus use much of the same evidence Lyell and Darwin would consider uniformitarian to argue for catastrophism and God's plan. In the conclusion to his *Geology* the usually diffident Dana, awed by the grandeur of all that he had seen and studied, let himself go and asserted that, despite all the differences and irregularities in nature, the earth was, after all, 'the result of a single plan of development.' Later, Darwinian evolution would have the same muted impact on Dana's thought.

After the completion of his Wilkes Expedition report on geology in 1849, Dana must have felt both pleased and exhausted. At the age of thirty-six he had already accomplished far more than most geologists did in a lifetime, and he probably needed rest. But relaxation did not suit his temperament, and he turned immediately again to mineralogy. He prepared the important third edition of his *System of Mineralogy* and pursued several current controversies, which at last promised to bring chemistry and crystallography closer together. One typical controversy concerned the 'polymeric isomorphism' of Thomas Scheerer, who thought that the differences betwen the hydrous and the anhydrous forms of cordierite (now considered to be $(Mg,Fe)_2 Al_4Si_5O_{18}$) could be explained as a substitution of three 'atoms' of water for one of magnesium oxide. At first this suggestion had seemed plausible, for such complex substitutions were becoming increasingly acceptable in the late 1840s, but Dana, Haidinger, and Rammelsberg finally rejected the idea by determining that Scheerer's aspasiolite was a pseudomorph and not an isomorph of cordierite.[23] Dana then went beyond Scheerer's theory and demonstrated that the atomic volumes of true isomorphs were roughly constant, but the theoretical significance of this similarity was not understood in the days before Cannizarro made the modern distinction between atoms and molecules.[24]

Dana's third edition also reflected the growing feeling that chemistry and crystallography were at last coming together. He rejected the long-held Mohsian natural historical system of classification, adopted tentatively a modified chemical plan, and included in an appendix the fully chemical plan of Berzelius, which Dana had first studied in the 1830s. Dana realized that his dramatic shift from one system to another could be considered inconsistent on his part, and to offset this criticism he made in his preface his oft-quoted remark: 'To change is always seeming fickleness. But not to change with the advance of science, is worse; it is persistence in error.' Unlike Dana, the European followers of Mohs had a far more difficult time in adjusting to the 1850s. Adolf

Kenngott of Vienna published in 1853 *Das Mohs'sche Mineralsystem, dem gegen wärtigen Standpunkte der Wissenschaft gemäss*, in which he disguised many of the new ideas as merely adjustments of the old system, but even then he was sharply criticized as being untrue to the master. In Europe, where traditions were stronger than in America, one had to be much more subtle about the change which Dana could proclaim so openly.

After this work in mineralogy, Dana returned in 1850 for the final time to his Wilkes Expedition labors. Perhaps he had left the Crustacea until last because of the poor condition of the specimens (due to a number of accidents), the difficulties of their classification, or, as he had written Redfield in 1839, his weaker interest in them. Although better studied than the zoophytes, the class was likewise a miscellaneous one. Again Dana had difficulty finding a basis for classification, since many of the animals seemed to lack hearts or stomachs, a deficiency that ruled out the use of the circulatory or digestive systems in classification. But Dana thought that they all had something of a head and therefore a nervous system. In fact, Henri Milne-Edwards had identified twenty-one essential segments in the head-thorax combination of the Crustacea. As Dana examined his specimens, which yielded over 500 new species, he found that as he went 'higher' in the gradation, more of the segments belonged to the head than to the thorax. The animals became increasingly centralized or 'cephalized,' with a higher 'concentration of force' in the head. He agreed that other animals such as insects might not follow quite the same laws as the Crustacea, although in the end, 'they must exemplify beyond doubt, the fundamental idea at the basis of those laws.' Cephalization appealed to his persistent ideas of unity, 'concentration of force,' and plans of development, and seemed to be still more evidence of the hand of the Creator. Once again Dana thought he had discovered one of the higher laws of nature. The idea had a broad appeal and was taken up by O. C. Marsh in paleontology and W J McGee in anthropology, but it has since been dismissed as a 'fanciful conclusion.'[25] It has been replaced by a greater stress on the degree of specialization of function rather than just physiological centralization.

Dana also went to considerable effort in his *Crustacea* to collect information on their geographical distribution in terms of ocean currents and water temperatures. In particular he wished to determine whether the species had been created locally or whether they had migrated to their present locations. He found that similar species did exist under similar ecological conditions, and in one case the identical species existed in both Japan and the Mediterranean Sea. He suggested the possibility of migration but rejected it rather hastily on the grounds that ocean currents would not explain it. He greatly preferred the idea of separate creations, even for identical species, and even went so far as to insist that 'this, in fact, becomes the only admissable view.' Dana must have been aware of the theological implications of the alternative view that two separate species might somehow have modified from one original form, and perhaps his orthodoxy explains his unusual rigidity and readiness to reject it as a possibility. In any case, Dana's labor on the *Crustacea* was a monumental one, and the final report, completed in 1852, filled over 1,600 pages in two volumes. With it Dana completed his ten-year involvement with the Wilkes Expedition reports. Undoubtedly he and those around him felt an immense sense of accomplishment and relief at their completion. They had been one of the major intellectual forces in his life; but in retrospect, perhaps because of the philosophical orientation of his work in mineralogy and of the conservative religious atmosphere in New Haven in the mid-nineteenth century, these massive volumes cast disappointingly little light on the emerging question of the transmutation of species. Dana, who had shown surprising openness, flexibility, and courage in breaking with the orthodoxy in mineralogy in 1850, refused only two years later to consider seriously the various kinds of evidence which suggested that traditional views of animal species might also bear reinterpretation.

After his achievements in the early 1850s Dana was typically in great haste to prepare still another edition, the fourth, of his *System of Mineralogy*. New works by Kenngott, Rammelsberg, Gustav Rose, Franz von Kobell, and others since 1850 indicated that the rigorously chemical system of Berzelius, which Dana had included in an appendix to the third edition but not used in the text, was the proper one, and Dana was anxious to make the correction. The revision, however, required such extensive changes in the text that Dana felt that he was writing a new work rather than editing an old one. It was to be Dana's last edition of his distinguished *System*. He issued semiannual supplements until 1859, when he could no longer carry on. George J. Brush, a former student of Dana who became a professor of metallurgy at the Sheffield Scientific School, and later Dana's son Edward Salisbury Dana took over the supplements and edited later editions of the *System*. The work is still the standard reference in mineralogy and is revised periodically by a team of prominent mineralogists.

After the completion of his latest work in mineralogy in 1854,

Dana embarked on the most public part of his career. With hindsight
we can see that it was unfortunate he did so much all at once, for in the
end it led to a collapse and shortened his period of usefulness. But for
about five years Dana was in the forefront of the major activities and
controversies of the day.

Elected president of the American Association for the Advancement of Science in 1854, Dana delivered an address entitled 'On
American Geological History' at the annual meeting in Providence in
August 1855. The speech epitomized Dana's religious, catastrophist,
and nationalistic views of geology. Citing the extensive work of
American investigators, Dana outlined the history of the North American continent from the Lower Silurian Age on through the Devonian,
Carboniferous, Jurassic, Cretaceous, Tertiary, and Post-Tertiary periods. Dana found evidence of long periods of oscillations in the earth's
crust followed by shorter periods of violent mountain building which
he attributed to contractions acting 'under Divine direction.' He also
reminded his assembled colleagues that the geology of North America
was much more simple and sublime than that of Europe and much
more suited to demonstrating the truths of creation. American geology
alone revealed God's plan of development, the detection of which Dana
thought, was the highest work of the geologist.[26]

Although Dana believed that geology should and could illuminate
religion—that geologists could interpret the Bible and should be
religious—he was not willing to extend reciprocal privileges to clergymen inadequately trained in geology. When such amateurs undertook
to interpret the rocks around them, or to express opinions on geological truths, or even worse, to criticize the personal character of certain
geologists, Dana, a leader and spokesman for his young profession,
endured such criticisms with difficulty. But when such unqualified
critics went even further and asserted that there was a 'conflict' between
Genesis and geology, or favored the developmental hypothesis to
which Dana had grown increasingly opposed, Dana, the man who
prided himself on having discovered God's plan of creation for the
animal kingdom and North America, if not the whole earth, bristled
with rage. Thus when in 1855 Tayler Lewis, a classicist at Union
College, wrote in his *Six Days of Creation* that science and religion
conflicted in their interpretation of Genesis, that the personal integrity
of several prominent geologists was in doubt and, worst of all, that
transmutation of species might be acceptable under certain conditions,
Dana felt compelled to respond. Several of his closest associates—
Professor Silliman, Arnold Guyot, Louis Agassiz, and Benjamin

Peirce—urged him on. Agassiz and Peirce felt that 'old fogies,' untrained in geology, had too long hindered the advance of science with their reactionary ideas of orthodoxy; Silliman and Guyot fervently wished for a new champion to defend the harmony of science and religion that they had always upheld, and would devote so much of their lives to supporting. In 1856 and 1857, in a series of four articles on 'Science and the Bible' in the *Bibliotheca Sacra*, a leading religious magazine, Dana battled Lewis by trying to show that science and religion were in complete harmony, or at least did not conflict, even though the actual connection might on occasion be beyond the mind of man. Dana's tone was quite emotional, like that of a man under attack, and he and Lewis hurled the epithet 'infidel' back and forth. Dana, who was usually so careful to be dispassionate in disputes and so anxious to avoid controversy, threw himself emotionally into this one, which struck at the very root of his being. Dana felt at the time that he had gotten the best of the argument, but opinion since then has been mixed.[27]

Perhaps the most extensive statement Dana ever made of his scientific philosophy was his 'Thoughts on Species' which he read at the AAAS meeting in Montreal in 1857. The views expressed were the culmination of his long interest in species, concentration of force, the unity of nature, the plan of development, and the use of analogies. The address also demonstrated quite explicitly the strong influence that mineralogy had had on his work and from which he had absorbed his idealistic approach to science. In the address Dana explicitly defined species as centers of force, that is, crystallization and attraction in mineral species and vital force in organic species. Mineralogical species were known to be fixed, and though there were frequent intermixtures, they differed only in discrete units. 'This being true for inorganic nature,' Dana reasoned, 'it is necessarily the law for all nature, for the ideas that pervade the universe are not ideas of contrariety but of unity and universality beneath and through diversity.'[28] Although species were in one sense 'permanent,' Dana recognized that they might also vary. In fact Dana acknowledged that variation frequently occurred. But species had definite limits, which were implanted in the type-idea of the species to guard its purity; the chemical Law of Multiple Proportions, which limited the possible combinations of minerals, was one such example. In working out this definition of species, Dana must have been gratified that he had been able to uncover another part of God's plan for the cosmos in the beautiful concept of species. Dana had been working with the concept for over twenty years, and now at last he had arrived at a congenial philosophical definition of it. He seemed finally to have received a full and consistent explanation of nature's unity and diversity. It was from this pinnacle that Dana would later try to come to grips with Darwinian evolution.

Dana was now, at the age of forty-four, at the top of his profession and his career. He had completed his massive volumes in classification, but he was busier than ever. In February 1856 he had taken up his professorial duties as one of the successors to the retiring Professor Silliman. Since then he had found that the daily lectures took more time than expected and frequently occupied his whole morning. He felt somewhat pressured, since he was also trying to prepare the mineralogical supplements to his *System*, run a fund drive for the Yale Scientific School, and edit the *American Journal of Science*. All together it was a heavy load, even for a man of Dana's abilities.

Although Dana had not been involved in the creation of the Yale Analytical Laboratory in 1846, he had taken charge of its affairs after the death of John Pitkin Norton in 1852. Dana chose John Addison Porter as Norton's successor and strongly urged Benjamin Silliman, Jr. to return from Louisville to help carry on the school. By 1856 Dana, the two Sillimans, and Daniel Coit Gilman, Herrick's successor as Yale College librarian, had decided that the school must have approximately $150,000 in the next few years for new professorships and a laboratory, if it were ever to become the center of science they desired. Dana became the leading spokesman for the school in the ensuing fund drive and filled the role Benjamin Silliman might have a decade earlier. He wrote the *Proposed Plan for a Complete Organization of the School of Science, Connected with Yale College* (1856) and delivered an address on 'Science and the Scientific Schools' to Yale College alumni in August 1856. How effective Dana's appeals were is hard to determine, but by 1860 the school had attracted almost the full amount from the local philanthropist Joseph E. Sheffield, the father-in-law of John Addison Porter.[29]

When in 1846 they became co-editors-in-chief of the *American Journal of Science*, Dana and Silliman, Jr. also succeeded Professor Silliman in still another role. The frequent absences of 'Young Ben' from New Haven meant, however, that the responsibility for the six issues per year usually fell upon Dana alone. Despite the additions of Wolcott Gibbs, Louis Agassiz, and Asa Gray to the editorial staff in the early 1850s, Dana continued to carry most of the burden of the *Journal*'s correspondence and editorial policy. This job also entailed settling the numerous professional squabbles of the 1850s. Dana always felt a sense of relief when he had put one more issue of the *Journal* into the mail and was very anxious to have Silliman, Jr. back in New Haven for advice and counsel.[30]

One of the most vehement quarrels of the 1850s took place in 1858–59 over Jules Marcou's *Geology of North America*, a book published in Zurich. Since Marcou overlooked much recent work on American geology and provided a highly inaccurate map, Dana criticized the work severely in a review in the November 1858 issue of the *Journal*. As always, Dana was concerned for America's reputation abroad and anxious lest foreign scientists judge American geology by this book so readily accessible to them. Dana's critical words, however, offended Marcou's friend Louis Agassiz, who sent Dana a strong rebuttal for inclusion in the next issue. When Dana resisted on the grounds that Agassiz had admitted not having read the book, Agassiz threatened to resign from the *Journal* if the defense did not appear. Dana, quite disturbed at his friend's turning on him in this way, compromised by letting the rebuttal appear and adding his own counterstatement in the January 1859 issue. In March, Marcou responded with a pamphlet, also published in Zurich, entitled *A Reply to the Criticisms of James D. Dana*, which the editors of the *Journal* (minus Agassiz who had left for Europe) responded to in the July issue by correcting some inaccuracies. They also expressed the conciliatory hope that if Agassiz had seen the pamphlet, he would have agreed with them, and they insisted that the dispute had not interrupted the usually 'cordial intercourse' between Agassiz and Dana.[31] It may have done more than that, however.

While the dispute with Marcou was still raging, Dana suffered a grievous personal loss in the unexpected death of his closest brother George at Utica in June 1859. On top of his heavy duties and professional tensions, this sudden blow staggered Dana. After a two-week visit to Utica in July, Dana returned to New Haven in such a state that two doctors recommended immediate rest, abstention from all work and excitements, and plenty of fresh air and exercise. The enforced leisure was difficult for a man like Dana, as his wife Henrietta wrote a cousin in August 1859: 'For a busy man to be systematically idle, and yet not have the time hang heavy is quite a problem.'[32] When he had shown little improvement two months later, the doctors recommended an extended tour of Europe. But the therapy was not effective, and when the couple returned ten months later, Dana had still not recovered. He was, however, sufficiently improved to be able to lead college prayers, one of his favorite duties. He seemed to be regaining his health slowly, but the death of his two youngest children, James Silliman Dana (age eight) and Harriet Trumbull Dana (age four), in a diphtheria epidemic in August 1861, was a great sorrow for both parents and a serious setback for Dana. Little Hattie was a particularly unfortunate loss, since she had been a great source of joy to her mother in the early days of James Sr.'s illness. After this double tragedy Dana recovered very slowly. He would never again be in robust health and after 1859 led a restricted life. At times he had relapses and could do no work for months. At other times he could teach his classes and work three to four hours per day. Yet even on this reduced regimen, Dana managed to 'concentrate his force' and to produce an average of three to four papers per year and to write or revise a book every other year for the next thirty-five years. It is startling to contemplate how much he might have accomplished had he been blessed with better health for this period of time.

Chief among Dana's publications after 1860 was his textbook, the *Manual of Geology*, which appeared in 1862, although almost all of it had been written before his 1859 collapse. Based on his Yale College lectures and his 1855 presidential address to the AAAS, it demonstrated Dana's conviction that the North American continent presented the simplest example of geological forces at work. The book traced American geology through the ages, describing each in turn with its characteristic strata, flora, and fauna. The *Manual* was therefore both vast in its scope and abundant in its geological and paleontological detail. The book was exceedingly popular, going through four editions in Dana's lifetime, and becoming one of the standard college textbooks for the next forty years. It was Dana's most influential work. If he had written nothing else, this book alone would have left his imprint on two generations of post–Civil War American geologists and mining engineers.

The later editions of the *Manual* also provide some of the few available clues as to Dana's reaction and gradual acceptance of Darwinian evolution in the 1870s and early 1880s. When he published the first edition in 1862, Dana had still not read the *Origin of Species*. In the second edition of 1874 he modified his views to allow for some continuity of species between catastrophes. He still balked, however, as one might have expected, at the gaps in the geological record and at the lack of an explanation for the actual 'origin' of new species, feeling instead that the evidence for continuity between generations far outweighed that for change. By 1883 when the third edition of the *Manual* had appeared and Dana was preparing a set of special lectures on evolution, it was clear he had accepted with reservations most of Darwinian evolution and was verging on Neo-Lamarckianism. He accepted the role of natural selection in modifying species, but not as the sole agent of change, and attributed more than Darwin to the influence of the environment, use and disuse of parts, and the inheritance of acquired characteristics. Like his friend Arnold Guyot, Dana also exempted human development from natural selection and retained a place for a God who could now direct evolution. Dana thus could not free himself totally from conservative religious influences, but by the 1880s he had changed his position from that of a 'modified catastrophist' to that of a 'modified Darwinian.'[33]

Dana's breakdown in 1859 thus did not put an end to his scientific development. Nor did his withdrawal from activity on the *Journal* end his influence in the politics of science. He was by the mid-1860s firmly established as America's preeminent geologist, and a letter from Dana long remained an important recommendation for a job on a state or federal geological survey. In the 1870s his influence may even have increased as his students Clarence King and O. C. Marsh performed important new work in the American West and rose to positions of national importance. At home in New Haven, Dana must have rejoiced in their exploits and achievements, as Silliman had rejoiced in Dana's own achievements forty years before.

Dana came to Yale in 1830 after Silliman had single-handedly started a tradition there in geology and mineralogy. By dint of 'ingenuity, industry + perseverance,' the facilities at Yale, and the experience of serving in the Wilkes Expedition, Dana was able to expand greatly on what had been known in Silliman's time and to raise natural science at Yale to even greater heights. Although much of his work was in classification, Dana was always seeking unifying principles beneath nature's diversity. He was, like Silliman, a devout Christian who considered it the greatest work of the geologist to uncover God's plan in nature. In the 1850s, when Silliman retired after his long career at Yale, his son, Benjamin Silliman Jr., and son-in-law, Dana, carried on after him—in Yale College, at the *Journal,* and with the Scientific School. Although Dana's public career was cut short by his breakdown in 1859, he continued his scientific work into the 1880s and 1890s, exhibiting much stoicism and Christian fortitude in the face of adversity. Silliman might well have been proud of such a son-in-law— there certainly were no others like him.

NOTES

[1]The denigration of naturalists is a constant theme in the history of American science, perhaps most forcefully presented in George Daniels' controversial *American Science in the Age of Jackson.*

2 Gilman, *Dana*, p. 14.

3 Asa Gray to Dana, 30 April and 1 May 1833, Dana Family Papers. Dana had had an earlier interest in botany (Dana to Father and Mother, 16 June 1825, Dana Family Papers).

4 'Professor Dana's Inaugural Discourse as Silliman Professor of Geology in Yale College,' *Am. J. Educ.*, 1855–56, *1*, 641–642.

5 Silliman [to Capt. Ballard], 1 February 1833, Dana Family Papers.

6 The best biography of Herrick I have found is Thacher, *Sketch of the Life of Edward C. Herrick*.

7 Dana to E. C. Herrick, 8 April and 21 April 1834, Herrick Papers. Herrick eventually published their findings alone while Dana was away on the Wilkes Expedition in 'A Brief Preliminary Account of the Hessian Fly and Its Parasites,' *Am. J. Sci*, 1841, *41*, 153–158.

8 Louis V. Pirsson, 'Biographical Memoir of James Dwight Dana, 1813–1895,' *Biogr. Mem. natn. Acad. Sci.*, 1919, *9*, 47. This obituary and Rice, 'Geology of James Dwight Dana,' in *Problems of American Geology*, pp. 1–42 are the best summaries of Dana's scientific work that I have seen.

9 *Am. J. Sci.*, 1835, *28*, 250–262. He later 'relinquished' it in the preface to his *System of Mineralogy* of 1837.

10 Gilman, *Dana*, pp. 38–41 and 344–347.

11 Dana to Silliman, 29 December 1834 and Dana to Father, 13 April 1835, Dana Family Papers.

12 *Am. J. Sci.*, 1836, *30*, 275–300.

13 Details of the expedition are provided in Gilman, *Dana*, ch. 5; D. Tyler, *Wilkes Expedition*; Bixby, *Forgotten Voyage*; Dupree, *Science in the Federal Government*, pp. 56–61; Reingold, *Science in Nineteenth Century America*, pp. 108–126; Ann Mozley, 'James Dwight Dana in New South Wales,' *Proc. Roy. Soc. N. S. Wales*, 1964, *97*, 185–191.

14 Haidinger, *Handbuch der Bestimmenden Mineralogie*, pp. xiii, 454, 458, 463; Rammelsberg, *Zweites Supplement zu dem Handwörtenbuch des Chemischen Theils der Mineralogie*, p. vi.

15 See Millhauser, *Just Before Darwin*; and Dupree, *Gray*, pp. 148 and 230.

16 The Danas were in Philadelphia seeing the *Zoophytes* through the press in October through December 1845. Their letters home to the Sillimans in the Silliman Family Papers offer one of the few glimpses of the young couple in the 1840s.

17 *Am. J. Sci.*, 1847, *4*, 364–385.

18 'Idea of an Atom, Suggested by the Phenomena of Weight and Temperature,' *Am. J. Sci.*, 1845, *48*, 352–368.

19 Gilman, *Dana*, pp. 209–210.

20 Dana to W. C. Redfield, 24 June 1839, Redfield Papers.

21 'On the Volcanoes of the Moon,' *Am. J. Sci.*, 1846, 2nd ser. *2*, 335–355; 'On the Origin of Continents,' *Am. J. Sci.*, 1847, *3*, 94–100; 'Geological Results of the Earth's Contraction in Consequence of Cooling,' *Am. J. Sci.*, 1847, *3*, 176–188; 'Origin of the Grand Outline Features of the Earth,' *Am. J. Sci.*, 1847, *3*, 381–398; 'A General Review of

the Geological Effects of the Earth's Cooling from a State of Igneous Fusion,' *Am. J. Sci.*, 1847, *4*, 88–92.

[22] Phillip Lawrence, 'Edward Hitchcock: The Christian Geologist,' *Proc. Am. phil. Soc.*, 1972, *116*, 21–34; and Stanley M. Guralnick, 'Geology and Religion Before Darwin: The Case of Edward Hitchcock, Theologian and Geologist (1793–1864),' *Isis*, 1972, *63*, 529–543.

[23] Rammelsberg, *Drittes Supplement*, pp. 7–8, 20–21; *Viertes Supplement*, pp. v–xiii.

[24] 'On the Isomorphism and Atomic Volume of some Minerals,' *Am. J. Sci.*, 1850, *9*, 220–245.

[25] Haller, *Outcasts from Evolution*, p. 102; and William N. Rice, 'Geology of James Dwight Dana,' in *Problems of American Geology*, p. 5.

[26] *Am. J. Sci.*, 1856, *22*, 305–349.

[27] Dana to Peirce, 7 July 1856, Peirce Papers; Morgan Sherwood, 'Genesis, Evolution, and Geology in America Before Darwin: The Dana-Lewis Controversy, 1856–57,' in Schneer, *History of Geology*, pp. 305–316; Tayler Lewis to Dana, 13 March 1871, Dana Family Papers, indicates there was a later rapprochement.

[28] *Am. J. Sci.*, 1857, *24*, 308.

[29] The Yale Scientific School in the 1850s is discussed in Rossiter, *The Emergence of Agricultural Science*, ch. 7.

[30] Dana's three letters to Silliman, Jr. in October–December 1852 and George J. Brush's to Silliman, Jr. 30 January 1853, all in Silliman Family Papers, show what need Dana had for a close associate at Yale.

[31] Dupree, *Gray*, pp. 256–257 and Lurie, *Agassiz*, pp. 271–275.

[32] Henrietta Silliman Dana to Harriet Silliman Trumbull, 20 August 1859, Brush Family Papers. Hattie Trumbull, a cousin of Mrs. Dana, later married George J. Brush. She was Mrs. Dana's confidante about James's illness, and Henrietta wrote her from Europe more than she did the family on Hillhouse Avenue. 'I haven't written all this home and wouldn't to anyone but you—but it is a great relief—*you* know—to say out what one thinks sometimes.' 28 November 1859, Florence.

[33] See William F. Sanford, Jr., 'Dana and Darwinism,' *J. Hist. Ideas*, 1965, *26*, 531–546 for a more complete discussion. Dana's good friend Arnold Guyot underwent a similar development between 1860 and 1880 and may have been a strong influence on Dana. See Dana, 'Memoir of Arnold Guyot, 1807–1884,' *Biogr. Mem. natn. Acad. Sci.*, 1886, *2*, 309–347, esp. p. 334.

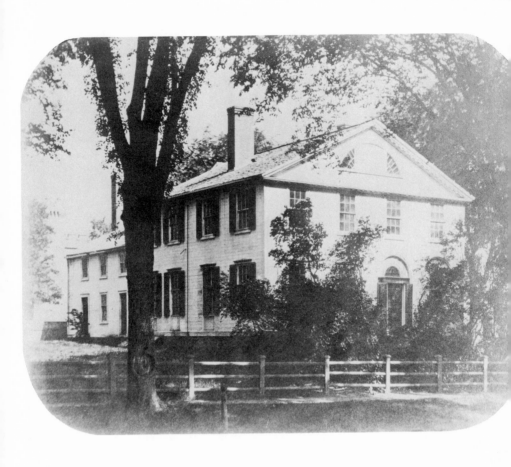

The School of Applied Chemistry at Yale from 1847 to 1852, the former house of President Day.

The Rise of the
Yale School of Applied Chemistry
(1845-1856)

LOUIS I. KUSLAN

ON 19 AUGUST 1846, the Yale College Corporation approved two new professorships in applied science. John Pitkin Norton, then but twenty-four years of age, was named professor of agricultural chemistry and of vegetable and animal physiology, and Benjamin Silliman, Jr. was elected professor of practical chemistry. Both men were extraordinarily well qualified for their positions. Norton's farm upbringing, his extensive study with both Benjamin Silliman, Sr. and Jr., with John W. F. Johnston in Scotland and Gerardus J. Mulder in Holland, and his missionary zeal for advancing the science of agriculture made him one of the best qualified persons in the United States to teach agricultural science even though he was not a college graduate. Benjamin Silliman, Jr., who had been well prepared at Yale by his famous father, had early shown great ability as a chemist, geologist, and teacher of the sciences.

These two young men, with the strong support of Benjamin Silliman, Sr., had persuaded the conservative Yale College faculty that the professorships were needed, and that, at almost no cost to the college, Yale could become a leader in meeting the demands of an emerging technological society.[1] From the college they rented the unused house in which President Day had lived, and, with some assistance from the college, converted it into a laboratory. Despite their hopes of ready donations from public spirited citizens, the two professors found that little money was available for maintainance. Student tuition could defray only a fraction of the cost and they were forced to use their own personal resources to purchase equipment. Some additional income, however, was derived from the commercial chemical analyses their students performed in their laboratory training.

Even though the School of Applied Chemistry, the name Silliman & Norton coined, was formally part of the Department of Philosophy and the Arts, inaugurated at Yale in 1847, the school's relationship with Yale College was informal. For some years, most students in the school had no direct connection with the college, although some were Yale College graduates or undergraduates. Although more than one

was interviewed on arrival by President Woolsey, they were neither
required to be college graduates, nor to satisfy entrance requirements.
They needed only express an interest in practical scientific study, and
were allowed to come and go each term as they wished.

The intent of the two founders of the School of Applied Chemistry
was simply to encourage the discovery of scientific principles and their
application to the practical arts, including agriculture, through research and instruction. They sought to unite science and man's daily
living for the benefit of both. During the five years in which John
Pitkin Norton directed the school, the major emphasis was on instruction in analytical chemistry, scientific agriculture, and geology. The
specific responsibility of Benjamin Silliman, Jr.—to apply chemistry to
the practical arts and particularly to manufacturing—languished and
was then abandoned for some years when, in 1849, Silliman took a
much more lucrative position in the Medical Department of the
University of Louisville.

The real instructional core of the scientific school was the laboratory and the informality of the curriculum contrasted strikingly with
the curriculum of Yale College. Formal courses of lectures were offered,
nevertheless. Benjamin Silliman, Jr. taught the first lecture course in
the new school in the fall of 1847. Lecturing from twelve to one o'clock
on elementary chemistry, he delivered a total of forty lectures. In the
winter term Norton gave lectures in agricultural science at the rate of
four a week for two months.[2] In the third term of 1847–48, Silliman
presented his lectures on applied chemistry and mineralogy, followed
by six weeks of geology. Denison Olmsted's excellent Yale College
lectures in natural philosophy were open to members of the Department of Philosophy and the Arts upon payment of a small fee. This
class, which began in the middle of the first term, met twice each week
for most of the year. In addition, Olmsted's lectures on astronomy and
meteorology were scheduled each day in the second term for seven
weeks, and for fifteen dollars students were permitted to attend Benjamin Silliman, Sr.'s famous chemical lectures.[3]

The beginning chemistry textbook was Benjamin Silliman, Jr.'s
First Principles of Chemistry, first published in 1847. This well-known
book was a veritable encyclopedia of elementary chemistry, for it
treated all fields of chemistry then known in a thorough, descriptive,
nonmathematical way. In it Silliman, Jr. took great pains to describe
within the limits of available space the applications of chemistry to the
practical arts, and it seems to have been admirably designed for his
course. In addition to his students' attendance at lectures, he expected
regular recitations on both his lectures and the textbook. Laboratory

work, too, was required, for Young Ben was not satisfied, as his father had been, to teach through lecture and demonstration alone.[4] Chemists were made at laboratory benches, not the lecture hall.

Norton at first required that his classes in agriculture read J.W.F. Johnston's *Lectures on Agricultural Chemistry and Geology* but when his book *Elements of Scientific Agriculture* was published in 1850, it naturally became his text.[5] Although not as experienced a teacher as his colleague, he too demonstrated important scientific principles but required less laboratory work. This was so probably because the majority of his students were interested farmers and not potential chemists. Norton was proud of the way in which he had planned his agricultural chemistry course. As he said, his lectures were 'perfectly intelligible to persons entirely unacquainted with chemistry, quite a number of those who propose attending the present course having never studied the subject at all. I bring in only so much chemistry as is necessary [and] explain everything new.'[6]

Farmers who were interested in learning some general principles of scientific agriculture, illustrated by specific examples, and in making 'simple examinations and analyses of soils and minerals' were invited to take the 'farmer's course.' No preparation was necessary since farmers could begin at the beginning as had 'the farmers who have hitherto attended . . . [and] have expressed their satisfaction and great interest.'[7] The course was available for the modest fee of $35 for tuition and $2.50 per week for room and board.

In addition to introductory courses, instruction was available in qualitative and quantitative analyses, the aspects of chemistry that soon dominated the curriculum. To make ends meet, the two young instructors sought to enroll as many students as possible. Had it not been for the continual investment of their own funds, the struggling school would have had to close soon after it was begun. The awareness of this struggle is evident in one of Norton's letters to J. W. F. Johnston:

> I have no salary nor any reason to expect one and my whole earnings in any one year since my coming here have not amounted to one half of my expenses, for the remainder I am obliged to be dependent upon my father. Before coming here and since that time I have had offers in connection with other situations that would have rendered me independent at once; I have preferred to remain here because I thought it the point from which I could do the most good.[8]

To inquiries about costs, Norton would answer that students should enroll for any length of time—a term, a month, or 'any time you think proper and pursue just such studies as you think fit.'[9] In reply to one inquiry, Silliman wrote: 'We have a class just now forming in Fresenius Chemical Analysis part first and another in part Second [quantitative analysis]. Should you decide to come it would be a good time to begin now. Our catalogue is now in the press and should you report yourself as coming we shall be happy to add your name to our list.'[10] How could anyone resist the lure of the low fee of $20 a month for the course in analytical chemistry, a fee which included reagents, glassware, and the use of excellent analytical balances?[11]

Norton relied heavily on advertising, and spent much time in answering inquiries from potential students. These answers explained the benefits of the special kind of firsthand instruction he supervised in the Yale laboratory. To a young teacher who asked for guidance in studying analytical chemistry at home, Norton was most discouraging. The necessary apparatus, he said, would cost at least $300, and the untutored analyst would soon be confronted with many insuperable difficulties. Norton's advice was that the writer save his money, then come to Yale for a few months each year for two or three years to work in the laboratory. In this way, 'You would make more progress in three months than you could in a whole year alone.'[12] John D. Easter, the recipient of this advice, heeded Norton's suggestion and a few years later received the Ph.D. degree in chemistry at Heidelberg University under Robert Bunsen.

Despite Norton's unrestrained enthusiasm for agricultural chemistry, laboratory instruction in this field, as distinguished from the regular work in analytical chemistry, was not heavily patronized. George Weyman, one of the original group of Ph.B. degree recipients in 1852, scorned the agricultural chemists he knew at Yale:

> At the end of last term we turned out 2 graduates in this course. They were supposed to be able to analyze soils, marl, etc. after a study of about 2 months. Just about two or three weeks before they left, I found the one who was considered to be the brightest of the two, testing for Cl by [silver nitrate] in a HCl solution and when I told him it would give a precipitate alone he doubted my word and said it did not. . . . These individuals go out now as students of Yale Analyt. Lab. It certainly will not do us much good.[13]

Norton's lectures and recitations in agricultural science were well attended by from twenty to forty young farmers in each class. Many of them had been attracted by heavy advertising campaigns; their fathers were often forward-looking men who believed that science might well have something to offer them. Norton's continual success in attracting large groups of students to his agricultural lectures was the result of his unusual blending of field experience in agriculture with theoretical and laboratory science. As he himself said:

> If I make one mistake and they [the farmers] catch me in it, they will remember it longer and talk over it more, than twenty instances of success. There is nothing that an old practical farmer will chuckle over with so much satisfaction as the detection of one whom he considers a theorist, in some blunder. In the first class that I taught in New Haven, I discovered, during my recitations, that some of the farmer boys were setting traps for me by asking the reasons for certain practical methods of proceedings. If they could have made me go into a scientific explanation of something which was to be referred to more common place or common sense reasons, they would have been highly satisfied.[14]

Norton's lectures obviously formed his book, which reads like a series of classroom lectures. He sought in its 208 pages 'to furnish a complete sketch of scientific agriculture, in plain and intelligible language; accompanied by as many details and explanations as deemed desirable in a purely elementary work.'[15] About one quarter of the book focuses on husbandry, pure agriculture, and the improvement of crops and farming practices. The remainder explains the scientific principles which underly agriculture. It interweaves chemistry, geology, agronomy, botany, physiology, and anatomy with progressive farming practices, both local and foreign. Professor Norton tried hard to fulfill his goal of giving his course of lectures 'such a character as to attract and interest that large class of farmers who know little or nothing about chemistry—to show them the proper connection of science with their pursuits, and to invite them to a course of study and reflection, calculated not only to improve their minds but to benefit them in the practical operation of their business.'[16]

If laboratory instruction in agricultural chemistry suffered while the agricultural lectures flourished, the laboratory was reasonably well filled with those who came to learn experimental chemistry. Some, like William H. Brewer, wanted to know how to perform soil analyses because 'at that time it was believed that the causes of the fertility of soils had been discovered and a remedy for barrenness provided. It was only necessary to analyze the soils, see what ingredients they lacked, apply them, and the problem was solved.'[17] Others, such as Samuel W. Johnson, came because they wanted to become professional chemists.

Even though in the laboratory there were no formal examinations for these young men, they worked hard. There were no requirements except to make something of themselves, a challenge which generated an aura of endeavor and fellowship. George Weyman, for example, wrote, after returning to New Haven from vacation in 1851: 'The old lab feels quite natural and comfortable now as cold weather comes on. It is pleasant to stand around the old sandbath, to look at your warm precipitates, etc. It was but yesterday that Blake, Weld, Craw and I stood by the old "bath" and talked of bygones. . . .'[18] Another student reminisced that 'No one knows the charm, which binds him to a laboratory and a set of students all enthusiastically working in the same glorious science.'[19]

William Brewer soon discovered that his daily life encompassed much more than soil analyses. On his arrival on Saturday, 21 October 1848, he visited President Woolsey and Professor Silliman, Sr. On Monday, he purchased his books, mainly chemistries, and visited the laboratory.[20] On Tuesday, he was 'appointed to recite the next day, washed my aparatus [sic] and arranged table ready for use.'[21] On Wednesday, he recited general chemistry to Silliman, Jr., and was shown some general laboratory techniques. On 11 November, only three weeks after his arrival, he 'commenced the analysis of the hundred bottles,' a graded series of qualitative analytical unknowns. Following the outline of qualitative analysis as customarily practiced at the University of Giessen, and turning to such authorities as Gmelin, Gustav Rose, and Jacob Berzelius, Brewer crept along with little help from his fellow students.[22]

On 21 November, Benjamin Silliman, Jr. began lecturing on mineralogy, and the class embarked on a number of field trips in order to collect specimens. Weekdays were reserved for the laboratory. Saturdays, unless an especially urgent analysis was on hand, were reserved for field trips. On 17 March 1849, Brewer was accompanied on a field trip by Mason C. Weld, David Hubbard, George Brush, William P. Blake, William S. Hillyer, and 'an academic.' The following week Silliman, Jr. took 'nearly all the students from the laboratory' to the Bristol (Ct.) copper mine where Ludwig Stadtmuller, a former student at the laboratory, was an official. They frequently returned to this mine. On 7 April they 'visited the serpentine quarries . . . [with] nearly all the students from the laboratory and several [Yale College] seniors, the excursion geological as well as mineralogical.'[23] Joseph Willett summed up these trips: 'You . . . miss the old mineralogical tramps. They were glorious evenings! Striding away 2 to 5 miles—breaking serpentine, chiselling out asbestos—Eating oysters along the beach—or climbing West Rock. The such will never come again.'[24]

The young scientists also botanized extensively, exchanging duplicates with friends far and near. Mason Weld and Ludwig Stadtmuller on one of their excursions collected more than 200 species and '4 times as many plants' within a few hours.[25]

There has been some consensus, presumably originating with Lounsbury, that students in the School of Applied Chemistry were isolated from Yale College.[26] This does not seem to have been completely true. Brewer and his colleagues, for example, were interested in many aspects of Yale College life, such as the 'Burial of Euclid.' They often attended the lectures of visiting dignitaries, and Brewer frequently referred to Yale College students who participated in field trips and in laboratory studies.

In his diary Brewer demonstrated that he was at Yale for a very special reason. However, he was not under great pressure until the end of his study in the spring of 1850. Then he wrote with obvious relief that he had 'finished my calculations on analyses and prepared to go home. Have been very busy for some time past to finish some analyses before the close of the term. Just finished with my calculations this afternoon.'[27] Though busy in the laboratory, he managed to find time to row and fish with his friends, including Professor Norton, and to visit in Connecticut and elsewhere. During the winter vacation of 1849–50, Brewer visited Chilton's and Doremus's laboratories in New York City, attended a meeting of the Brooklyn Natural History Society, and a lecture by Dr. Draper at the Van Rensselaer Institute. A few days later, he visited the Medical College at Albany, the New York State Geological rooms, and the lecture on agricultural science which he described as beautiful and interesting. He also visited Professor Emmons's laboratory and the State Normal School in Albany.

By 1849, Brewer had become sufficiently able as an analyst to undertake complete analyses of specimens sent to the laboratory for examination. The following are examples of his tasks:[28]

June, 1849	Gypsum specimens from Cayuga County, New York and from Nova Scotia
July, 1849	Limestone specimens from Sing Sing, New York
Feb., 1850	Hudsonite from Orange County, New York
Feb., 1850	Determination of nitrogen in white fish, dried for manure
Feb., 1850	Examination of an intestinal calculus
Apr., 1850	Soil from Arkansas
Aug., 1850	Meteorite from Salt River, Kentucky

Of the eighty analyses entered in the laboratory record in the four and one-half years the record was kept (many analyses are not recorded in this volume), the largest number, fifteen, were completed by George J. Brush; Brewer completed ten; Benjamin Silliman, Jr. was responsible for two, not including his analyses of Goodyear's rubber samples; Norton completed two and collaborated on one; twenty students are recorded as having completed one or more analyses.

The laboratory was the most important aspect in the practical education of the analytical chemist. Commercial analyses undertaken at the request of individuals brought from $5 to $25, a rate which both Norton and Silliman considered much below their true value. Even though the laboratory lost money, the experience gained was indispensable to the students. There was a vast difference between routine analytical testing of fabricated 'unknowns' and the real problems brought to the lab from the nonacademic world.

Within a year or two Norton realized that many of his students, capable chemists though they were, were deficient in certain vital branches of education. Most of them remained in the school for only a short time, but by 1850 at least a dozen had been in attendance for a year or more, and several for nearly two years. A number of students were planning scientific study abroad. To prepare them properly, Norton required recitations in rhetoric each week as well as an essay on a scientific topic every two weeks.[29] The title of one of these essays was 'The Atmosphere in its adaptation to the wants of man.' Some students elected to study French and German, and a few took advanced mathematics at Yale College. One of these students remarked that his days had become so busy that he could go to bed no earlier than eleven o'clock in the evening, and was forced to be up by six o'clock in the morning in order to keep up with his work.[30]

Benjamin Silliman, Jr. maintained a connection with the School of Applied Chemistry for some time after he left in 1849 for the University of Louisville. He returned to New Haven periodically to visit his father and family, and taught at the school during the summer term. This arrangement soon became unsatisfactory, and in 1850 Norton bought out Silliman. In September 1850, Norton wrote a bitter letter to his colleague, complaining about Silliman's reputed criticism of Norton's 'parsimony' in purchasing chemicals, apparatus, and journals for the laboratory. Norton seems also to have been annoyed by reports that his 'co-ajutor' had sought to lure some of his laboratory students to Louisville.[31]

Young Ben strongly denied such double dealing; he was still, he said, a firm exponent and supporter of the school. 'My withdrawal and quasi-connection with the laboratory was I fear an injury to you— although I did or tried to do all in my power to prevent it.'[32] The time, however, was obviously right to sever their relationship, and he was now prepared to sell out his interest in the laboratory for $1,020. This offer was accepted in November 1850 by Norton who paid that sum for Silliman's 'stock, apparatus and outfit of the analytical laboratory.'[33]

The two had earlier attempted to develop mutually agreeable arrangements for the laboratory. Shortly before Silliman left New Haven for Louisville, he had offered to take 'one quarter of the *net* profits of the *year* after [Norton] paying all expenses.' His share was to include his services for the summer term of the School of Applied Chemistry, the use of the Silliman name and 'influence' which was obviously valuable, and the use of his half of the school's equipment and supplies. In the circumstances and in view of his needs, he believed that he would be much better off to sell out completely, 'But I feel too much interest in your success, and that of the school to do anything which would in the least injure either.'[34]

Despite the occasional grumbling about shortages of reagents and journals, students seem to have been satisfied with the limited resources of the laboratory. They knew that they would have to study in Germany if they were to complete their education as chemists. A number did so. They accepted the laboratory with its limitations as a stepping stone to new careers, even though they often looked ahead apprehensively to the future. They were much more inclined to grumble because Norton spent too little time in the laboratory than because they lacked platinum crucibles. Brush, for example, complained: 'Norton we know is a competent teacher, but he does not work with students. Under these circumstances do we not need reform?'[35] And some months earlier after the 'tyrannical' first assistant, Henry Wurtz, had been fired, Weyman rejoiced: 'We almost love [Norton] who now spends more time in the laboratory and is interested in everything which went on.'[36]

Norton's interest in directing his own students was short lived. He soon became immersed in the newly projected university in Albany, New York. Early in 1852 he began to spend only three days a week at his post in New Haven, even though there were twenty-four students then at work in the laboratory.[37] William Craw, the first assistant, remarked after Norton's death in 1852 that Professor John Addison Porter, Norton's successor, spent a great deal of time in the laboratory with the students, 'an improvement over the old system.'[38]

Norton was obviously torn between the School of Applied Chemistry, which demanded time, the proposed university, and his enthusiasm for proselytizing among farmers for the reform of agriculture and agricultural education.[39] He was not a chemist by choice. He was, rather, an agricultural reformer who chose agricultural chemistry and improved education as the road to reform, and it was because of this mission that his young chemists suffered.

Benjamin Silliman, Jr., on the other hand, seems to have been much better suited to direct the laboratory. He was a son of Yale. He had initiated and maintained a small research and teaching laboratory of his own, and he was not committed to a missionary role. He was also a skilled teacher. One of his students once said that he 'rather preferred hearing [Young Ben] than his father. He gave a more complete view of his subject and digressed very little to tell stories or mention "My friend, Dr. Hare"' (though it is only fair to add that the Yale College Class of 1849 thought it 'very dull sport to hear "Young Ben."'[40])

At Louisville, Silliman was considered to be the most popular of lecturers. He was experienced in preparing demonstrations, having served as the chief assistant to his father for a decade, and having ordered and maintained the chemicals and supplies in his father's laboratory. He failed, however, to fulfill his responsibility to the laboratory when at Yale by not giving it his full time. He continued, for example, to help his father prepare the demonstrations, hear the seniors recite, and substitute when Silliman, Sr. was absent from his lectures in chemistry and geology. He spent many more hours as editor of the *American Journal of Science* and took charge of much of its correspondence. Spurred on by the needs of a large and growing family, he added to his schedule a variety of such tasks as steamship boiler inspections, school lectures, and writing his very popular chemistry textbook.[41] He was one of the founders of the New Haven Gas Company, a business which soon returned excellent dividends to its stockholders. His house was the first residence in New Haven to be illuminated by gaslight. Benjamin Silliman, Jr., therefore, was too busy to give all the time which was needed for the management of the school. It seems quite clear that neither of the two directors, Silliman, Jr. or J. P. Norton, fully exerted the kind of educational leadership of which they were capable.

Soon after Silliman announced that he was leaving for Louisville, Norton sought a new partner. He wrote O. Wolcott Gibbs, then teaching at the Free Academy in New York City, describing the opportunities in New Haven. Gibbs visited New Haven to discuss Norton's proposition, but even though Gibbs professed interest in becoming 'entirely independent of college routine and of all the annoyances of a subjection to trustees and committees,' he rejected Norton's blandishments: 'With the influence of the College to assist us and the facilities of instruction which by uniting our forces we should be able to afford we could beyond question in my opinion make this the leading chemical school of the country. . . .'[42]

After all, Norton continued, 'A person of much inferior qualifications' could fill Gibbs's place in New York, and Gibbs would be free at Yale to follow any system of instruction he chose. What was more, both Norton and Silliman were certain that they could easily raise ten thousand dollars to support the laboratory and that the college would give land for a 'beautiful laboratory.' There was at Yale a sufficiency of assistants 'who are willing and anxious to work two or three years for their instruction.'[43]

Norton's appeal was liberally sprinkled with references to Gibbs's 'patriotism,' and to the 'rare opportunity' in New Haven. Would Gibbs come if he were given a full year in order to arrange his affairs? Gibbs did *not* come, and the reason he gave is instructive. He confessed that he was a Unitarian, and he was afraid that New Haveners would be hostile to him for this reason. As a result, he would not dare to come unless he were completely reassured on this point. Reassurance was obviously not strong enough, nor could Norton conceal from Gibbs the fact that the School of Applied Chemistry faced an uncertain future. There was still no money for salaries, and the few dollars from fees were insufficient to support a man with a family.[44]

Gibbs suggested Josiah D. Whitney in his place, but Norton's doubts concerning Whitney were reinforced by 'several of our gentlemen here [New Haven].'[45] Few chemists in the United States met Norton's requirements, but Dr. Gibbs was one of them. Norton continued to pursue Gibbs, and in July 1852, a few months before his death, he urged James Dwight Dana to persuade President Woolsey to appoint Gibbs to the chemistry professorship at the next meeting of the Yale Corporation.[46] This plea also failed.

To fill the gap temporarily, Silliman, Jr. and Norton were forced to appoint as a laboratory assistant Henry Erni, a young Swiss protégé of Louis Agassiz. His duties were to take charge of analyses of 'ores, minerals and etc. [sic] to be entrusted to him,' to direct the laboratory, and to help its students. 'It is indispensable,' Silliman wrote, 'that he who fills this place should well understand chemical inorganic analysis—as much as in general organic analysis.'[47]

Erni, who was hired in October 1849, was named Chief or First Assistant, at $400 a year, and was given an unfurnished room on the second floor of the laboratory building to serve as a bedroom. He was encouraged by Norton to eke out his modest salary with lectures in botany and other aspects of natural history.[48]

Norton was still trying to lure a first rate chemist to New Haven,

and discussed his school with J. W. F. Johnston, his former teacher in
Scotland, on the occasion of the latter's tour of the United States. For a
few months there seemed to be a real possibility that Johnston would
join Norton in New Haven, especially since 'Johnston was somewhat
unpopular at home.'[49] But in the end Johnston returned to Scotland,
embittered and critical of the United States in general, and unhappy
with Norton in particular.

Henry Erni remained at New Haven for a year, and was succeeded
by Henry Wurtz, a brilliant but contentious young chemist and
mineralogist. Wurtz attained some fame in later life through his
research in several scientific and engineering fields, and particularly in
illuminating gas chemistry as a coworker with Benjamin Silliman, Jr.
Wurtz also remained only a year. He was thoroughly disliked by the
students who resented his dictatorial and supercilious attitude toward
them. Weyman once quoted Wurtz as saying that 'It was very difficult
for a young chemist to get along with a parcel of . . . mean and
ungentlemanly . . . students.'[50] The situation became so intense at one
point that the students threatened to pack up and leave unless Wurtz
was dismissed. He left reluctantly, and Norton, who was aware that
Wurtz was an excellent chemist, was just as reluctant to force his
departure, but he had no other choice.[51]

The first assistantship was now bestowed on William J. Craw, a
steady if unsophisticated chemist, who had been one of the first
students enrolled in the laboratory in 1847. Brush described him in
these words:

> Craw is a good natured conscientious, easy and in the yankee sense clever
> [man], but you know as well as I that there is not a particle of fire or
> enthusiasm in him. Give him a good process and he will make a good
> analysis. I trust more to results made by Craw by a good process than
> almost any person I am acquainted with.[52]

This choice was not acclaimed by Craw's fellows, however. They
had hoped that a man with a different training and with new ideas
would be hired.[53] Nevertheless, Craw held the school together in the
many difficult days that followed, as Norton first spent half of each
week lecturing in the new university at Albany, and then became
hopelessly ill.

Norton's illness was first diagnosed as a heart condition, but it
proved to be tuberculosis. In March 1852 he left New Haven for Florida
to recuperate, having 'given up all idea of lecturing for a year at
least.'[54] Since Norton had six lectures still to deliver in New Haven,
Mason C. Weld, one of his students (and a relative), lectured in his

place. Weld was frantically busy at this time since he was himself studying advanced geology, mineralogy, and German and was also assisting Benjamin Silliman, Sr. with Silliman's Yale College chemistry lectures. Weld and Craw together handled Norton's correspondence and the finances of the laboratory.[55]

The students, hoping for the return of their teacher, responded to every rumor of his good health, but Norton was not to recover.[56] During his return to New Haven from Florida, Norton fell ill with the measles at Washington, and in his already weakened condition, death came quickly. He died in Farmington, Connecticut at the home of his father, John Treadwell Norton, on 5 September 1852. In his will he left the contents of his laboratory to Yale College with the request that the college allow the laboratory to continue; his two best balances he left to Weld and Craw.

There was little his students could say or do at the end except to express their grief:

> That modest, amiable, lovely countenance, with manner so gentle and frank, and a readiness to assist every one, we can never forget! It seems that it would not be unmanly to weep for Professor Norton, where there was so much to love and so little to censure.[57]

The number of students who came for an extended period of instruction, that is, one or more terms, fluctuated from year to year. Beginning with the six registered in 1847, the number rose to ten in 1848, fell to nine in 1849, then increased to twenty-one in 1850-51, and to twenty-four in the winter of 1851-52. In the summer term of 1852 only a handful of four registered compared to fifteen the summer before. This was to be expected, because the laboratory had fallen on hard times with Norton's illness. These few, however, were optimistic about the future because they expected 'a great many seniors [would be] coming in.'[58] In the 1852-53 academic year, there were twenty-five chemists, including a number with baccalaureate or even Master of Arts degrees, of whom a few were from Yale College. Many of them were transfers from Brown University at Providence, Rhode Island attracted to New Haven along with Prof. John Addison Porter who had been appointed to Norton's post.

In 1850 New Haven and Yale College were host to the annual meeting of the American Association for the Advancement of Science, an event which aroused great interest in the community. Of a total of 460 members in 1849, 15 were from New Haven. John P. Norton, Benjamin Silliman, Jr., and Denison Olmsted, Jr., a son of the Yale professor of natural philosophy, were members, and in 1850 twelve students were elected. Several participated actively in the meeting. William H. Brewer, for example, read a paper entitled 'Determination of Nitrogen in Two Varieties of Indian Corn' on which he had worked feverishly earlier in the year so that it would be finished in time.[59] When his work was criticized by Dr. Charles T. Jackson, John P. Norton spoke up for his protégé, arguing that Brewer's paper proved that 'ultimate' analysis was more important in agricultural chemistry than was 'proximate' analysis. Jonathan B. Bunce's paper. 'Analysis Relative to the Economical Value of Anthracite Coal Ashes' received the combined attention of Robert E. Rogers, O. Wolcott Gibbs, Eben N. Horsford, T. Sterry Hunt, William P. Blake, Benjamin Silliman, Sr., Henry Wurtz, and Franklin Bache, truly a distinguished group of commentators.[60]

Many of the students planned to study with the great European chemists, and a sizeable number realized this dream. John D. Easter, Edward Hungerford, George Weyman, Ezequiel Uricoechea, Francis Dakin, and William Hillyer were enrolled from 1852 to 1855 at Wöhler's laboratory in Göttingen, where Uricoechea and Weyman received the Ph.D. Uricoechea had earlier taken the M.D. degree at Yale. George J. Brush, William H. Brewer, Mason C. Weld, Samuel W. Johnson, and Ogden N. Rood traveled to Munich to work with Liebig who, however, was no longer active in the laboratory. Instead they worked with Pettenkofer and Von Kobell, both well-known analysts. None of this group remained long enough to complete the Ph.D. degree. Nearly all studied with at least one other well-known European chemist, generally in Germany, but sometimes in England or France.

Brush, Johnson, and Brewer eventually returned to the Yale Scientific School, as the scientific-engineering segment of the Department of Philosophy and the Arts became known in 1854. Others, including some who had studied abroad and many who did not, continued in the sciences. Some of them, however, saw no future in scientific research. Brush was shocked when Jonathan Bunce left the laboratory to enter business with his father. 'The rascal deserves a thrashing,' he wrote. 'I expected better things of him. I loved Bunce and I hoped he loved science enough to make her his espoused.'[61] Others, like Matthew G. Wing, David L. Hubbard, William Hillyer, and John Crooke were forced to leave because of ill health, financial difficulties, or because they were attracted to other careers. Hillyer, for example, became a successful lawyer in Indiana.

Their anxiety about the future was expressed by Samuel W. Johnson who wrote that 'the only way for a poor chemist to make his fortune was [to marry a rich wife].'[62] Craw ruefully noted that 'the

demand for the services of a chemist with a remuneration sufficient to
fairly pay for these services are in reality but few and far between.'[63]
Craw, however, was not the dynamic and creative chemist that his
friends Brewer, Brush, and Johnson were. He suffered from severe
personality problems which impaired his ability to work effectively
with people.

Brush, so disappointed by Bunce's renunciation of science, was an
ardent proselytizer for science. He sought to take science to the hinterlands:

> We all feel that it would be very pleasant to live in New Haven,
> Philadelphia, or Boston where scientific men are plenty, but we shall all of
> us probably find our mistake; we must go out into the unscientific portions
> of our country and there raise up science, by so doing, we shall render a
> much more acceptable service to science than if we were the propounders
> of some abstruse theory or the discoverers of new elements, planets, or
> comets.[64]

Brush, however, did not remain long in the hinterlands, although
a few of his friends were to find satisfying careers there. Most of them,
like Henry Erni, who left his first assistantship for what he thought was
a better position in Tennessee, were unhappy because they were far
from congenial friends with whom they could live science.[65] As Joseph
Willet in Georgia wrote:

> At Yale, we had those of the same advancement . . . with whom we
> could discuss points, and show our ignorance and broach our conjectures
> with perfect freedom: and then, after we had become tangled in a knotty
> subject, we had professors to whom we could more gravely propose
> our difficulties and have the knot undone in a more scientific manner
> than our Gordian way of cutting them . . . it is almost discouraging
> to go on excursions with no companion to sympathize in developing
> our curiosities.[66]

Norton often compared the opportunities at his little school with
those at the Lawrence Scientific School at Harvard. He believed that
only at Yale could a man receive 'a thorough course of instruction' in
practical farming.[67] To an inquiry about the value of study abroad, he
replied that J. W. F. Johnston's laboratory in Scotland was very
expensive, and, in any case, would soon be closed. There were one or
two laboratories in London where agricultural chemistry was taught,
but they were not worth the trip. The continental laboratories, he said,
were the

> best schools in the world for the study of . . . chemistry, but there is not
> much application to [agricultural] practice. . . . We have a number of

remarkably promising young men now with us. . . . It would be unbecoming in me to say anything in praise of the advantages here. I can only say that I am most anxious to diffuse knowledge on the subject of an improved agriculture and therefore of course use every means for the instruction of my students.[68]

Eben Horsford's laboratory at Harvard was much better equipped and financed, but 'I think it may fairly be said that we [at Yale] know more about the applications of chemistry to practical matters than they do at Harvard.'[69] Norton advised young men who asked about study in Europe to spend two years at Yale and then go abroad for a year of advanced work. This, he said, was 'cheapest and judging from my own experience the best course.'[70]

Norton radiated optimism about the future for the graduates of his school, an optimism which was, as we have seen, not shared by all his students. He often answered those who asked about employment in characteristic fashion:

I have not yet been able to fill more than two thirds of the applications that have been made to me for young men to fill responsible situations as instructors, assayers. . . . I know of no opening in a professional way so promising as that of the various affiliations of chemistry, more particularly those connected with agriculture.[71]

Benjamin Silliman, Jr. was similarly positive:

We would say that in our opinion the profession of a well informed chemist and mineralogist offers at present as many inducements as any other learned profession or art. The various applications of such knowledge to the arts and manufactures gives annually many desirable openings for persons who are properly qualified and agriculture and mining are also frequent sources of similar employment.[72]

The students worked long hours in the laboratory in order to make the most of their opportunity there. Those who had little money, a sizeable number, were naturally limited in their social activities. The others were more fortunate. Yale College was a major cultural center, and the members of the school took advantage of the lectures and concerts. When Jenny Lind's train passed through New Haven, they waited eagerly at the railroad station for a glimpse of the famous singer. They turned out to watch the football games between the college classes; they were aware of the activities of the various Yale societies and knew the names of those who were tapped. They attended the 'swarrys' given by President Woolsey for Yale College classes, and the evening parties given by the faculty and other prominent New

Haveners. The social life of a small inbred town like New Haven was unbelievably busy, with continual visiting for tea, for dinner, and for every conceivable occasion. The laboratory students took part in many more of these events than commentators on the early years of the school have allowed.[73]

Students who left the laboratory wrote to those who remained to ask the latest news of New Haven. Several returned to New Haven more than once to renew old friendships. They reminisced in the most sentimental way:

> I think that you cannot scare up such another crowd [as the laboratory group] in the U.S. large as it is. I have been going to school all my life since I was able to walk, mixed in with societies, clubs, and so forth, and never found their equal.[74]

In 1848 they organized the Berzelius Society which, for a number of years before it became a social fraternity, served as a forum for student discussion and for invited speakers. In addition to the scientific aspects of the society, a social purpose was served through the regular monthly evening suppers, held sometimes on Thursday, and other times on Saturday. The nature of their discussions is indicated by the titles of two of the papers read to the group: 'A Defense of Aerial Navigation,' and 'On the Relative Values of Fresenius and Will's Qualitative Analysis.' College students were encouraged to join. In 1851 at least two seniors and one sophomore were members, and there was an expectation of adding 'some more to our number from the Academical Department.'[75]

At the 16 February 1853 meeting they debated Denison Olmsted's theory of the formation of the aurora borealis. Craw commented that fourteen members, a larger number than usual, were present. In 1851 William H. Brewer sent the society fossil shells from Lancaster, New York and described in some detail the rock from which they had been taken. Mason Weld, the Berzelius Society secretary, informed Brewer that 'the Berzelian Society were highly pleased, interested, and instructed,' and that the members sought answers to these questions: 'Is this deposit now forming? Does it form rapidly? Is the surface water of the region highly charged with lime? Is the quantity of nitrogen and of phosphoric acid present sufficient to make the deposit of greater value than lime or gypsum?'[76]

Their relationship with Benjamin Silliman, Sr. was obviously excellent, for the grand old man of American science had consented to give a course of lectures in order to raise money for the society in 1852, but because of his ill health the plan was abandoned. 'As he is our main dependence,' Weyman lamented, 'we gave up without further deliberation.'[77]

Several of the laboratory regulars assisted Benjamin Silliman, Sr. in preparing and giving his lectures to the Yale College seniors after Silliman, Jr. had left New Haven. The elder Silliman noted that 'the last lecture [in his 1851 chemistry course] was given to the freezing of carbonic acid and mercury. The entire thing was entrusted to Mr. Weld aided by Mr. Blake and Mr. Craw of the Scientific Department and was entirely and beautifully successful.'[78] They had been helpful, as well, in 1849 and 1850. Brush, Brewer, and Erni had also served as assistants to the elder Silliman at one time or another. In 1850 Mason C. Weld was appointed assistant to Silliman. In one term he received $62.50 from the 'fees of ladies and gentlemen,' in addition to a stipend of $125.[79] Benjamin Silliman, Sr. always referred to Weld and his friends in the most complimentary of terms. He called Weld 'a young man considerably expert in Chemistry and altogether zealous devoted and amiable.'[80]

Although the chemistry students in the Department of Philosophy and the Arts had been admitted without examination, except for an interview with either Norton or Silliman, Jr. (and occasionally with President Woolsey), and as a matter of practice they elected from the curriculum only what they wished, they were supportive of a formal degree program. In 1847, the corporation had considered a degree program, but had postponed the matter for future consideration.[81]

By October 1851 the students began to campaign vigorously for the degree. George J. Brush was worried about what would happen unless the corporation instituted the degree and an organized curriculum:

> I am afraid the Laboratory in New Haven will go to the devil this winter if more exertion is not made to sustain it. . . . Norton . . . is obliged this winter to spend more than half his time in Albany and Craw is at the head of the Labt. Is it possible under such circumstances for the Labt. to succeed?
>
> Between ourselves the only way is for the Professor . . . to take hold with all his zeal and endeavor to inspire all his students with enthusiasm, to cultivate a high aim in science among them and at last have a diploma which can be procured only by a course of study for a certain length of time and then not till they have passed an examination.[82]

In November, Weyman wrote to Brewer to announce the happy tidings:

> The faculty have just decided concerning our degrees. The first degrees will begin next commencement, and the qualifications are these. Eighteen

months spent in the Lab and of course implying a knowledge of Analytical Chemistry—one modern language;—and one other science, Geology, Botany, Mineralogy—for instance. I inquired of Prof. Norton if such as you and Brush that had gone away could be candidates; he answered that you certainly could. We therefore hope that you will become one of the class of '52. You know enough of Analytical Chemistry, of Botany or Geology and you could by that time perfect yourself in French or German. That degree will be PhB [Bachelor of Philosophy] or SB [Bachelor of Science]. When you write inform me if you cannot possibly join us. We expect to have Weld, Craw, Johnson, Bunce, Blake, Brush, Olmstead, three unknown to you, yourself, and myself. So you see we have a large class, larger than they ever will have hereafter I expect. What a glorious and happy time we would have if we could all come together once after taking our laurel wreath to sit down and talk over our good old times when we were students—now the 'Alumni of the Scientific Department.'[83]

A committee composed of President Woolsey, Benjamin Silliman, Jr., and John Pitkin Norton decided on 6 November 1851 that a proper degree would be awarded to those members of the Department of Philosophy and the Arts who completed the requirements that had been proposed by Norton acting in collaboration with Benjamin Silliman, Sr. and James Dwight Dana. On 19 December 1851 this committee formalized the regulations pertaining to the degree of Bachelor of Philosophy, a title for which Norton had argued strongly.[84]

Weyman added other details. The language examination would be 'nominal,' he said, since President Woolsey had agreed with Norton that the students would have too little time to prepare for a rigorous language examination. 'As to chem, geology, etc., I would like to see any one of us stuck, particularly on analyt. chem. . . . My own private opinion is that every one of us will get through.'[85]

The decision to award the degree stemmed from Professor Norton's petition of 19 December 1850 which, supported by Professors Edward Salisbury, Denison Olmsted, Benjamin Silliman, Sr., and James Dwight Dana, requested the Prudential Committee of the college to consider 'the expediency of connecting some degree or diploma with the termination of a certain course of study in the Philosophical Department of this College.'[86] Norton even suggested that this degree be like the 'German Doctor of Philosophy,' but the time was obviously not right for the latter proposal.

In 1851 Norton addressed a second petition to the president and the corporation of the college considerably extending his ideas. This petition was signed by Professors Noah Porter, W. A. Larned, J. L.

Kingsley, Thomas Thacher, and James Hadley. In it, Norton referred to the high quality of the students in his department. He discussed the value of a degree program in lengthening the period of study and in improving the education of the students. Furthermore, the degree would provide the struggling department with additional support from the college. Norton now suggested the degree 'Bachelor of Philosophy' or 'some other honorary title as may to your wisdom seem preferable.'[87]

The corporation delayed action at this time, although there was a continuing discussion within the faculty of the merits of the degree. President Woolsey was not favorably inclined. Most of the faculty, however, were regarded as being supportive of degrees for the 'fourth department.' In a third memo, Norton suggested certain rules:

> Students who have been members of this school for a period of time not less than two years, for at least 18 months of which they must have been actually present and taking full courses shall be entitled to present themselves for examination in not less than three distinct branches of Natural Science and Modern Languages.
>
> Students in Chemistry to be examined in General, Elementary, and Analytical Chemistry, Organic and Inorganic, both Qualitative and Quantitative. This examination is to be according to the character of the course each one has pursued, either in the general applications and theories of Chemistry, or as applied to the Arts and Agriculture.
>
> Students in Mineralogy to be examined on the use of the Blowpipe, the general determination characteristics of minerals and the laws of their classification.
>
> Students in Geology to be examined as to the relative order and age of geological formations, the laws of stratification, and of igneous action, the occurrence of fossil remains, and the economical bearings of the science.
>
> Students in Botany to be examined on the classification of plants, the order of their distribution, the means of determination, and their general value for food or for manufacturing purposes.
>
> Students in German or French to be examined as to their knowledge of the construction of either of these languages and to be able to translate readily from the ordinary scientific works.
>
> The text books from which the examination is conducted to be selected by the teachers in the several branches.
>
> Those students who shall pass satisfactory examinations in any three of the above studies and who shall have complied with the foregoing regulations as to time of membership in the department shall be entitled to the degree in Philosophy.[88]

On 27 July 1852 the corporation at last voted to accept the new degree, adding that the graduates must be at least twenty-one years of age, and must pay a graduation fee equal to that imposed on the Bachelors of Arts and Laws.[89]

Their vote was anticipated because students were actually examined on 16 July 1852, a few days before the corporation acted. They were examined by Benjamin Silliman, Sr. in geology, by Benjamin Silliman, Jr. in chemistry, and by James Dwight Dana in mineralogy and botany. Craw, Brush, Brewer, Shepard, Blake, and Weyman, the first group, did well, although it was noted by Norton that Blake and Weyman had not performed quite as well as the others.[90]

On commencement day in 1852 these six young men of the Department of Philosophy and the Arts, who had been enrolled in the School of Applied Chemistry, were awarded the degree of Bachelor of Philosophy. They were, up to that time, the best prepared group of young chemists graduating from an institution of higher learning in the United States. All but Craw pursued successful scientific careers. Four later taught in colleges, three at Yale. Craw, because of serious illness, was forced to abandon the sciences soon after graduation.

It is not easy to assess the achievements of Norton and Silliman. During the two years in which Benjamin Silliman, Jr. was active, his many publications were primarily mineralogical analyses, contributions to the realm of the pure sciences with little relevance to the practical arts. Student research bore little relationship to the practical arts, although Jonathan Bunce's paper at the 1850 American Association for the Advancement of Science meeting was well received, and both Silliman, Jr. and Norton helped Goodyear in his rubber research.

The years of Norton's leadership from 1848 to 1852 were successful in drawing the attention of farmers to the value of chemistry to agriculture, but there was little pure research in agricultural science. Although farmers often turned to the laboratory for analyses of soils or fertilizers, and Norton gave them practical advice to enable them to make the best use of the analyses, this was not research and his students were well aware that some vital element was missing. In 1852 one of them wrote, 'Such men as Profs. Norton, Silliman, Johnston, etc. are not qualified to advance this science [agriculture] rapidly—they are analysts, but not farmers.'[91] Silliman, Jr. and Norton were called 'analysts,' but even as analysts, students suggested that their work would have been much more valuable had they run comparative experiments on prepared and unprepared soils so that cause-and-effect conclusions might be drawn.

Norton would surely have been offended by this harsh judgment because he took great pride in his credentials as a working farmer. However, he lacked an experimental farm for testing his ideas, a deficiency of which he was well aware. In a speech to the New York State Agricultural Society in 1848, he had proposed the creation of an agricultural school to include an experimental department with three divisions:

> 1. A Chemical department, devoted to such investigations and researches in chemistry, as should lead to valuable practical results.
> 2. A Veterinary department, where the diseases of animals can find proper treatment, and where the qualities of various breeds should be ascertained.
> 3. A portion of the farm, on which to test the various questions discussed in the school and elsewhere, by cultivation.[92]

From the point of view of the practical arts, little was accomplished. The laboratory performed services for those who could pay for chemical analyses. Some contributions were made by the students and faculty to mineralogy, to organic chemical analyses, and to soil analyses. In the main, however, the laboratory was a teaching institution, and it was through the preparation of well-trained young chemists that the School of Applied Chemistry made its special contribution.

Even more important was the fact that in the few years in which Norton and Silliman, Jr. were in charge, they managed to establish the laboratory so securely that it survived Young Ben's departure and Norton's untimely death. They proved to the Yale Corporation, to the Yale faculty, and to their students that the school served an important purpose at Yale and was therefore entitled to a place in Yale education.

Much new information about the period after Norton's death has recently become available. Two new professors, the chemist John Addison Porter and the engineer William Augustus Norton, joined the staff. The Sillimans maintained their interest in the well-being of the school and its students, both in helping to appoint new faculty members and in raising money. Benjamin Silliman, Jr., who returned to Yale in 1854 to succeed his father as professor of chemistry, continued to hold a part-time teaching position in the Scientific School which was formed by the merger of the engineering and chemical schools of the Department of Philosophy and the Arts.[93]

In 1855 the two Sillimans secured the appointment of Samuel W. Johnson, one of the graduates in 1852, to the staff of the school. Late in 1854 or early in 1855 Johnson had written to the junior Silliman from Europe to seek a position as a laboratory assistant, but there was no opening because Professor Porter's brother, Charles, already occupied this position. Since Professor Porter was chiefly responsible for the laboratory, Silliman answered: 'It is not right for me to give you any encouragement, however much I should like to do so.'[94] He would, however, welcome Johnson to work in his own laboratory, 'the old college laby' which could be his 'chemical home.' At this time, early in 1855, Silliman, Jr. had not taken an active role in teaching in the Scientific School and stated: '[I] shall not do so until some change shall make it a sufficient foundation for *one* professor. To divide Prof. Porter's cherry could not be to confer any favor on him.'[95]

Again on 30 April 1855 Silliman, Jr. wrote Johnson with more encouraging news, urging him not to take a job elsewhere until the two of them could confer about the situation at Yale. Although Silliman's reason for optimism was not stated, it seems to have stemmed from certain 'important changes. . . . in the prospects of our School,' which could only have been John Addison Porter's engagement to Josephine Sheffield, one of Joseph Sheffield's daughters.[96] Sheffield, a wealthy and public-spirited man, was soon to become the school's benefactor and many interested New Haveners now anticipated 'an endowment completed and complete.'[97] Sheffield, writing in 1875, supplied partial confirmation for this speculation: 'My attention to the wants of the college was first excited after [Josephine] . . . was married to Prof. Porter (in 1855) who was then a Professor in the department of philosophy and the arts; and I think that before I went abroad, in 1856, I made a donation of 5 or 6000 dollars.'[98]

Both Silliman, Jr. and Brush (who had already been notified that he would be appointed professor of metallurgy, an appointment confirmed in July 1855) were anxious to secure Johnson. 'And now that Porter has something to live on (as I suppose he undoubtedly will have) the interests of the school will be shared more equally among the Profrs. and all will have a word to say about the *first* assistant.'[99] Brush soon had more news to report. Silliman, Jr. was busy trying to find a teaching position for Porter's brother, and the prospects were good that Johnson would soon be able to replace him. Brush quoted Silliman as saying that 'no effort of mine will be wanting to that end [to employ Johnson and to pay him a suitable salary].' He also quoted Dana that 'Porter would soon leave the Labt pretty much in [Johnson's] hands where [Brush] would like to see it.'[100]

Through an error of the corporation, Johnson was named first assistant in the analytical laboratory. He had been nominated by Silliman, Jr. and James Dwight Dana to an assistant professorship, and had been informed of this nomination by Silliman, Jr. in July 1855. Silliman had further stated that the salary for this professorship was to be $600 a year; Johnson was also entitled to a room in the college if he wished. Silliman, Jr. and John A. Porter personally guaranteed Johnson's salary if the school should become unable to pay it.[101] Johnson reluctantly accepted the first assistantship. Brush reminded him that 'Dana and Silliman feel the vital importance of having you remain, and are provoked beyond measure at the stupidity of the Corporation's blunder of not giving you the title they (the profrs) had intended. . . . You have no idea of what a high estimate they put upon your opinion.'[102] It is no wonder the corporation blundered since the 'conspirators' were addressing themselves almost entirely to the lesser position.

The corporation elevated young Johnson to a full professorship on 29 July 1856 after a year's service as first assistant, a promotion which was more than anyone had dared to hope for. Both Sillimans recommended Johnson to President Woolsey, urging upon him the importance of such an appointment and assuring him of Johnson's fitness for the position. They reminded Woolsey that they had known Johnson since 1848 as a student and assistant. The elder Silliman, in concluding his recommendation, said: 'Should Mr. Johnson be enlisted in the great enterprise of the Scientific School, I cannot doubt that his labors and influence will be fruitfully applied to promote the success of an Institution which appears to be regarded with decided and increasing favor by our intelligent fellow citizens.'[103]

The Sillimans continued to seek support for the school. Benjamin Silliman, Sr. was instrumental in the purchase in 1856 by Mr. Sheffield of certain property which was eventually donated to the school. A number of prominent gentlemen from Connecticut met in Silliman, Sr.'s home on 15 April 1856 to consider further development of a 'scientific and agricultural school,' a step which encouraged Sheffield all the more in his philanthropic and filial assistance.[104]

In 1856 the Sillimans participated in a memorable drive to raise money, when on 4 June the most distinguished citizens of the state were invited to hear James Dwight Dana speak on 'The Utility of Science.' The committee that arranged this gala occasion was headed by Benjamin Silliman, Jr.[105] An earlier printed appeal to interested citizens was signed by both Sillimans, President Woolsey, and the faculty members of the Scientific School.[106]

Benjamin Silliman, Sr., on the occasion of Joseph Sheffield's gift of a splendid building and a large endowment in 1860, wrote Sheffield at some length to thank him for his donations. In closing his touching and sentimental letter, he alluded to his long interest in the school:

I should not have presumed so much on your kindness had I not been gratified, more than I can express, by the happy progress of our truly good and useful institution under your auspices. As the original mover of this enterprize—and as its Sponsor on the Baptismal Font, I may be pardoned, I trust, for my freedom. . . .[107]

Sheffield, in his reply, acknowledged this devotion:

To you . . . who have labored for more than fifty years, under rather discouraging circumstances, to build up that important department, it must be particularly encouraging and gratifying to witness, in the evening of your days, an increasing interest in the institution on the part of your countrymen, and an appreciation of its value that will not only sustain it in its present usefulness, but carry it forward to perfection.[108]

The younger Silliman continued his association with the Sheffield Scientific School, although in a nominal way, until 1869, the year in which he submitted his resignation. That same year Charles W. Eliot, the new president of Harvard University, said:

Established in 1847 at a time when a thrill of aspirations and enthusiasm seems to have run through all the New England Colleges . . . [The Department of Philosophy and the Arts in Yale College] *is at once an epitome of the past history of scientific instruction in this country and a prophecy of its future.*[109]

Could there be a more fitting epitaph for the Sillimans and John Pitkin Norton?

NOTES

[1] Louis I. Kuslan, 'The Founding of the Yale School of Applied Chemistry,' *J. Hist. Med.*, 1969, *24*, 430-451. This paper describes the events leading up to the foundation of these professorships.

[2] *Cultivator*, 1847, *5*, 324-325; Norton, 'Lecture Notes,' Norton Papers.

[3] *Yale Coll. Cat.*, 1847-48, p. 43.

[4] Norton to R. Warner, 22 January 1850, 'Letter Press Book of the Yale Analytical Laboratory,' Sheffield Records.

[5] Norton to Prof. W. Kingsley, 10 January 1851, 'Letter Press Book of the Yale Analytical Laboratory,' Sheffield Records. The excellence of Norton's book is indicated by an unsigned review, probably by Henry Barnard:

The publishers have issued the 10th thousand of this admirable work, the production of a scholar of rare abilities and still rarer powers of adapting his great acquisitions to the wants of practical men. His early death is still widely lamented, but this volume and the various essays which at different times appeared from his pen, will for many years to come, remain as standard guides to those who are engaged in the honorable pursuits of agriculture. No one will be prejudiced against 'Book-Farming' who reads and practices the instructions of this volume.

Am. J. Educ., 1856, 2, 745.

6 Norton to R. Warner, 22 January 1850, 'Letter Press Book of the Yale Analytical Laboratory,' Sheffield Records.

7 Norton to R. Jones, 9 August 1849, 'Letter Press Book of the Yale Analytical Laboratory,' Sheffield Records.

8 Norton to J. W. F. Johnson, 9 December 1851, Norton Papers.

9 Norton to J. Whitman, 15 November 1849, 'Letter Press Book of the Yale Analytical Laboratory,' Sheffield Records.

10 Silliman, Jr. to Dr. Breed, 30 November 1848, 'Letter Press Book of the Yale Analytical Laboratory,' Sheffield Records.

11 Norton to J. Whitman, 15 November 1849, 'Letter Press Book of the Yale Analytical Laboratory,' Sheffield Records.

12 Norton to J. D. Easter, 11 November 1850, 'Letter Press Book of the Yale Analytical Laboratory,' Sheffield Records.

13 G. Weyman to Brewer, 19 April 1851, Brewer Papers.

14 Norton, 'Connection of Science With Agriculture,' *Proc. N. Y. St. agric. Soc.*, 1852, p. 175.

15 Norton, *Elements of Scientific Agriculture*, p. v.

16 *Cultivator*, 1847, 5, 324.

17 William H. Brewer, 'A Century of Connecticut Agriculture,' *Rep. Conn. St. Dep. Agric.*, 1895, 28, 36.

18 G. Weyman to Brewer, 5 November 1851, Brewer Papers.

19 Brewer, July 1850, Brewer Papers.

20 Brewer, 21 October 1848 in 1848–50 diary, Brewer Papers.

21 *Ibid.*, 24 October 1848.

22 *Ibid.*, November entries, 1848.

23 *Ibid.*

24 J. Willett to Brewer, 14 February 1850, Brewer Papers.

25 M. Weld to Brewer, 21 November 1851, Brewer Papers.

26 T. R. Lounsbury in Kingsley, *Yale College*, II, 106.

27 Brewer, 24 April 1850, in 1848–50 diary, Brewer Papers.

28 'Analytical Laboratory Record Book,' Sheffield Records.

29 Norton, 24 January 1851, diary, Norton Papers.

30 G. Weyman to Brewer, 28 November 1850, Brewer Papers.

31 Silliman, Jr. to Norton, 19 September 1850, Norton Papers.

32 *Ibid.*

33 Receipt given by Silliman, Jr. to Norton, 16 November 1850, Norton Papers.

34 Silliman, Jr. to Norton, 13 September 1849, Norton Papers.

35 G. Brush to Brewer, 19 November 1851, Brewer Papers.

36 G. Weyman to Brewer, 28 November 1850, Brewer Papers.

37 Norton to Dr. G. S. Henry, 14 February 1852, 'Letter Press Book of the Yale Analytical Laboratory,' Sheffield Records; Norton, November 1851-February 1852, diary, Norton Papers.

38 W. Craw to Brewer, 11 November 1852, Brewer Papers.

39 Norton frequently complained about his heavy schedule, yet he continued to take on additional duties. For example, in response to a plea from a publisher in Scotland that he undertake an American edition of a Scottish farming book, he said that to do it he would be forced to use much of the 'time which I ordinarily devote to my Laboratory duties of analysis and Instruction.' He accepted the chore, however. Norton to Robert Blackwood, 18 April 1848, 'Letter Press Book of the Yale Analytical Laboratory,' Sheffield Records.

40 E. Jarvis to Brewer, 30 November 1851, Brewer Papers.

41 Silliman, 'Personal Notices,' 10 November 1848 and 21 January 1849, Silliman Family Papers.

42 Norton to O. W. Gibbs, 7 June 1849, 'Letter Press Book of the Yale Analytical Laboratory,' Sheffield Records.

43 *Ibid.*

44 O. W. Gibbs to Norton, 21 June 1849, Norton Papers.

45 *Ibid.*

46 Norton to J. D. Dana, 29 July 1852, Norton Papers.

47 Silliman, Jr. to Henri Erni, 29 June 1849, 'Letter Press Book of the Yale Analytical Laboratory,' Sheffield Records.

48 Norton to H. Erni, 20 July 1849, 'Letter Press Book of the Yale Analytical Laboratory,' Sheffield Records; see also W. D. Miles and L. I. Kuslan, 'Washington's First Consulting Chemist, Henri Enri,' in Rosenberger, ed., *Columbia Historical Society*, pp. 160-161.

49 J. Willett to Brewer, 14 February 1850, Brewer Papers.

50 G. Weyman to Brewer, 28 November 1850, Brewer Papers.

51 Norton to Henry Wurtz, 16 April 1851, 'Letter Press Book of the Yale Analytical Laboratory,' Sheffield Records.

52 G. Brush to Brewer, 19 November 1851, Brewer Papers. Norton sought the advice of Benjamin Silliman, Sr., James Dwight Dana, and other Yale faculty members as to the qualifications of prospective faculty members and assistants. See also Norton's diary, 27 March 1851, Norton Papers.

53 G. Weyman to Brewer, 19 April 1851, Brewer Papers.

54 G. Weyman to Brewer, 30 March 1852, Brewer Papers.

55 W. Craw to L. Case, 7 April 1852, 'Letter Press Book of the Yale Analytical Laboratory,' Sheffield Records.

56 G. Brush to Brewer, 23 May 1852, Brewer Papers.

[57] G. Weyman to Brewer, 25 November 1852, Brewer Papers.

[58] G. Weyman to Brewer, June 1852, Brewer Papers.

[59] Brewer, 'Determination of Nitrogen in Two Varieties of Indian Corn,' *Proc. Am. Ass. Advmt Sci.*, 1851, pp. 386-389.

[60] J. B. Bunce, 'Analysis Relative to the Economical Value of Anthracite Coal Ashes,' *Proc. Am. Ass. Advmt Sci.*, 1851, pp. 213-215.

[61] G. Brush to Brewer, 19 November 1851, Brewer Papers.

[62] W. Craw to Brewer, 19 December 1852, Brewer Papers.

[63] W. Craw to Brewer, 17 February 1853, Brewer Papers.

[64] G. Brush to Brewer, 28 November 1852, Brewer Papers.

[65] Norton to Erni, 20 July 1849, 'Letter Press Book of the Yale Analytical Laboratory,' Sheffield Records.

[66] J. Willett to Brewer, 30 April 1852, Brewer Papers.

[67] Norton to unknown correspondent, 9 August 1849, 'Letter Press Book of the Yale Analytical Laboratory,' Sheffield Records.

[68] Norton to R. Howland, 11 July 1848, 'Letter Press Book of the Yale Analytical Laboratory,' Sheffield Records.

[69] *Ibid.*

[70] *Ibid.*

[71] Norton to Mr. Seabury, 26 November 1851, 'Letter Press Book of the Yale Analytical Laboratory,' Sheffield Records.

[72] Silliman, Jr. to W. Murray, 1 March 1848, 'Letter Press Book of the Yale Analytical Laboratory,' Sheffield Records.

[73] The letters, diaries and other contemporary accounts of student and faculty life at the school are filled with such social activities. See, for example, G. Weyman to Brewer, 22 January and 19 April 1851, Brewer Papers; also, Norton diaries for 1851 and 1852, Norton Papers; also Hadley, *Diary (1843-1852)*.

[74] G. Weyman to Brewer, 2 September 1852, Brewer Papers; also, J. Willett to Brewer, 24 September 1849, Brewer Papers.

[75] G. Weyman to Brewer, 28 November 1851, Brewer Papers.

[76] G. Weyman to Brewer, 5 March 1852, Brewer Papers.

[77] G. Weyman to Brewer, 5 June 1852, Brewer Papers.

[78] Silliman, 'Accounts of B. Silliman for Yale College Laboratory for 1850,' Silliman Family Papers.

[79] *Ibid.*

[80] Silliman, 'Personal Notices,' 2 October 1849, Silliman Family Papers.

[81] W. Larned, 'John Pitkin Norton,' in *Memorials of John Pitkin Norton*, p. 47.

[82] G. Brush to Brewer, 19 November 1851; W. Craw to Brewer, 12 December 1851, Brewer Papers.

[83] G. Weyman to Brewer, 5 November 1851, Brewer Papers.

[84] Norton to the President and Corporation of Yale College, undated, 1851, Sheffield Records; Norton, diary, 6 December and 19 December 1851, Norton Papers.

[85] G. Weyman to Brewer, June 1852, Brewer Papers.

[86] Norton to the Prudential Committee of Yale College, 19 December 1850, Sheffield Records.

[87] Norton to the President, Corporation and Fellows of Yale College, 1851, Sheffield Records. No action was taken at this time although there was a continuing discussion of the merits of the degree among the faculty. President Woolsey was reported as not being in favor, although most of the faculty were in favor of degrees for the 'fourth department.' See Hadley, *Diary (1843–1852)*, p. 269.

[88] 'Rules and Course of Study in the Philosophical School of Yale College,' unsigned but in Norton's hand, Sheffield Records.

[89] Larned (n. 81), p. 48.

[90] Norton, 16 July 1852, diary, Norton Papers.

[91] J. Willett to Brewer, 30 April 1852, Brewer Papers.

[92] *Proc. N. Y. St. agric. Soc.*, 1848, p. 608.

[93] Silliman, Jr. planned to teach introductory chemistry in the first term, mineralogy and technical chemistry in the second and third terms. Silliman, Jr. to Johnson, 2 July 1855, in Johnson, *From the Letter-Files*, p. 91.

[94] Silliman, Jr. to Johnson 27 February 1855, Johnson Manuscripts.

[95] *Ibid.* That financial matters for John A. Porter were difficult is clear from the letter of recommendation written for him by Benjamin Silliman, Sr. on 13 January 1854. The elder Silliman praised Porter and remarked that 'His separation from Y. C. would be regarded as a great loss to that Institution.' Silliman, 'Personal Notices,' 13 January 1854, Silliman Family Papers.

[96] Silliman, Jr. to Johnson, 30 April 1855, Johnson Manuscripts; G. Brush to Johnson, 12 April 1855, Johnson Manuscripts.

[97] G. Brush to Johnson, 12 April 1855, Johnson Manuscripts.

[98] Joseph Sheffield, 'Joseph Sheffield to His Son,' 17 March 1875, pp. 43–46, Sheffield Records.

[99] G. Brush to Johnson, 12 April 1855, Johnson Manuscripts.

[100] *Ibid.*, 13 May 1855.

[101] Silliman, Jr. to Johnson, 2 July 1855, in Johnson, *From the Letter-Files*, pp. 90–91.

[102] G. Brush to Johnson, undated but about December 1855, Johnson, *From the Letter-Files*, p. 93.

[103] Silliman, to President Woolsey, 26 July 1856, Sheffield Records.

[104] Chittenden, *Sheffield Scientific School*, II, 585–588.

[105] H. Farnham, *The Sheffield Scientific School*, Yale University Memorabilia Room.

[106] Woolsey, et al., *Appeal in Behalf of the Yale Scientific School*.

[107] Silliman to J. Sheffield, 19 October 1860, Sheffield Records.

[108] J. Sheffield to Silliman, Fisher, *Silliman*, II, 278.

[109] Eliot, 'The Sheffield Scientific School, As Seen by An Outside Observer,' in Yale College, Sheffield Scientific School. *Explanatory Statements for the Freshman*, pp. 26–27.

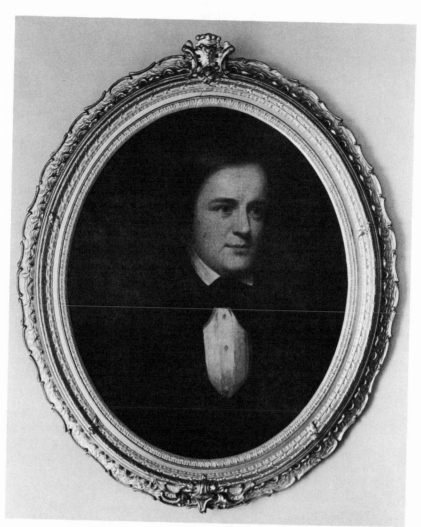

Benjamin Silliman, Jr., aet. 35.

Benjamin Silliman, Jr.:
The Second Silliman

LOUIS I. KUSLAN

BENJAMIN SILLIMAN, JR. (1816–85), although not exactly obscure, nevertheless lived for many years in the shadow of his father. He did not gain the respect and admiration which deluged the elder Silliman who knew himself to be both a true scientific pioneer and an acknowledged leader among American scientists. Because Benjamin Silliman, Jr. was deeply devoted to his father, the precious early years—so important in the making of a scientist of the highest level—were dissipated as he served his father's needs first and then attended to his own aspirations. Instead of perfecting himself in scientific research in Europe or in an apprenticeship to a good American scientist, the younger Silliman relied almost completely on self-instruction (except for what he learned directly from his father and other Yale mentors); and like so many who are self-taught, he exhibited surprising deficiencies in his training. Never once, however, did he give a sign of anger or rebellion against his father.

Josiah P. Cooke, referring to some events which marred Silliman's later years, said:

> If he sometimes made mistakes of judgment, they were the results of an over sanguine and trustful temperament, not sufficiently regulated by the caution which the training of a mining school and the life of a mining camp gives to those who have been bred to the profession of a mining engineer. Certainly, no one suffered from the consequences of his mistakes as greatly as himself.[1]

Although Benjamin Silliman, Jr. died some twenty years after his father, this biographical essay is focused on his career and his relationships with his father and the members of his father's circle while his father was alive. As a result his later career, which is perhaps the most fascinating and least known facet of his life, is treated in the most cursory fashion. White's excellent study, *Scientists in Conflict*, describes in detail certain aspects of the younger Silliman's later years, particularly Josiah Dwight Whitney's implacable enmity which darkened most of Silliman's days after his father's death. Because of the special focus of this essay, most of Silliman's business and research interests, his work at Yale, as well as his personal and social life, have not been examined, despite their considerable interest.

For the sake of variety, Benjamin Silliman, Sr. is referred to by that name, and as Benjamin Silliman, the elder Silliman, and Professor Silliman. Benjamin Silliman, Jr. is referred to as Benjamin Silliman, Jr., Silliman, Jr., Ben, Young Ben, the younger Silliman, or Silliman.

Young Ben's impetuosity, his faith, which was sometimes a simple gullibility, and his incredibly varied business and professional pursuits, blemished his work as a chemist and mineralogist and, to his great sorrow, affected his scientific and personal reputation.

Most of those who knew him well, however, would have agreed with Timothy Dwight, president of Yale from 1886 to 1899:

> Professor Silliman, the younger . . . had much of his father's geniality. He was kindly to all. The hospitality of his house was appreciated by every one who knew him. The winsomeness of his manners rendered him attractive. His readiness for conversation fitted him for social intercourse and made his companionship pleasant to his friends. The knowledge and information which he had gained in different lines, through his studies and his travels, he was ever willing to communicate to others and he was thus disposed to be helpful to them. In his temperament he was cheerful and sanguine. A certain roseate view of life seemed to place him apart in his thoughts and hopes from many around him who had, in their own opinion at least, a more just and sound estimate of things. There was something inspiring for him, no doubt, in this mental attitude, but it was attended at times by a possibility of disappointment. His courage and ardor, however, were unfailing, and he moved forward under their influence toward the end he had in view.[2]

That he was close to his father is clear. When he learned of his father's death, he unburdened his heart to his wife:

> The great fear I had from the commencement of my journey [to California in 1864] was that my dear old father might not remain until my return! This fear I have more or less clearly expressed to you several times. And now it is true! To have lost the pleasure of so many months of his love and counsel is something forever to be regretted—to have been deprived of the sad pleasure and duty of assisting by my presence in the last acts of devotion and filial piety leaves a blank which nothing can fill. I have however been spared perhaps some trials which were inseparable from seeing his decline and am permitted always to remember him as I ever knew him and last saw him—fresh, vigorous, with mental power and vitality unimpaired.—You know my meaning and what measure of consolation there is in it. Few men reach middle of life as I have done with *so* much cause for grateful memories to *both fathers* [a reference to Mrs. Silliman's father and to his] both now in Heaven.—I rejoice that my children knew him so well and enjoyed his love so much.[3]

Benjamin Silliman, Jr. was born on 4 December 1816, when his father was thirty-seven years of age. He was the fourth Silliman child and the first son to grow into maturity. Three brothers and a sister died at early ages. He early displayed scientific and practical interests. Of Benjamin, his father once wrote:

> If I have found occasion to confess myself a partial judge in the case of Mr. Hubbard and Mr. Dana what shall I say when my own son is the subject of my remarks. I might indeed name him [as] the successor of Mr. Dana and do no more.
>
> But it would be weak and foolish to laud him because he is a part of myself. It would be unjust indeed, for that reason, to withdraw from him his just due. I shall therefore treat him with Roman impartiality and describe him as he is.
>
> In early life, in his school boy days, he was not fond of the study of language particularly of Greek and Latin and therefore, after entering College, he did not take that stand to which his talents entitled him.
>
> From his earliest day, however, he manifested mechanical talents of a high order. He was not inclined to folly and he took great delight in visiting shops and manufactories not only to see but understand their curious processes. In two instances when he was missing from his school for several days together, it was found that in one instance it was to learn the art and mystery of forming the mould for the casting of iron and in another that of making hats. He had no propensity to engage in the follies of boys or to resort to improper places of amusement. . . .
>
> His love of mechanics was so strong and his talents in that line were so decided, that almost as soon as he had reached his teens I indulged him in the possession of tools of which he made so good use that a shop was fitted up for him in a wing of the house with ample conveniences including a lathe of iron constructed by himself and a furnace with bellows, anvil, etc. was added.
>
> In College he early discovered a love of Natural Science and of the mathematics and his mechanical training harmonized well with these more mature developments. During his College life he was of course familiar with the doings in the laboratory and he therefore very naturally passed into the situation of assistant as soon as he had finished his undergraduate course in 1837.
>
> He had become, in the mean time, a good writer, and was in all respects qualified for the place which he filled with ability and to my entire satisfaction during twelve years from 1837 to 1849 having served in the department more than twice as long as any one of his predecessors. Of course he became familiar with the sciences which we cultivated and he was able to lecture occasionally in my place in the college and in popular courses to the citizens of New Haven and other places. . . .
>
> His familiarity with tools, instruments and manipulations in addition to a knowledge of the sciences taught in the department qualified him to be an able and expert assistant and filial feeling was of course in

harmony with the obligations of public duty, having had so long a course
of experience with me.

He was therefore the more able to fulfill my wishes when I was absent
and to make all the requisite preparations of the experiments.[4]

The school to which Benjamin Silliman referred was the Hopkins
Grammar School in New Haven. Young Ben was surely not a
schoolboy paragon. He was well known for 'outrageous school pranks'
and for frequent truancies when he was said to 'run in and around the
alleys rather than get his lessons.'[5] He seems to have been a ringleader
in a violent schoolroom insurrection which ended only when the
leaders were vigorously 'cowhided' by trustee James L. Kingsley,
professor of classics at Yale College, in front of their fellows. The elder
Silliman who was not personally involved in this particular incident
was serving at the time as a trustee of the Hopkins Grammar School.
Young Ben 'liked to remind his listeners that four of the offenders
became ministers.'

There were few options for students at Yale College, and Ben
suffered through the traditional Yale curriculum of Latin, Greek,
rhetoric, etc., much to his later advantage as a lecturer and historian of
science. However, he also heard his father's lectures in chemistry,
geology, and mineralogy and Denison Olmsted's lectures in natural
philosophy.

As an undergraduate Ben was active in the Yale Natural History
Society and served for some time as secretary and treasurer. He was
especially successful in obtaining donations of rocks, minerals, and
fossils for the society both during and after his graduation from Yale.[6]

In addition, Ben assisted his father and, best of all, was often taken
along on Professor Silliman's frequent consulting visits to mines. In
1836, while yet a junior at Yale, he spent two months with his father
and a friend inspecting the Virginia gold mines. While visiting the
University of Virginia, he took advantage of the opportunity to attend
William B. Rogers's geology lectures.

When he graduated as a Bachelor of Arts in 1837, Benjamin
Silliman, Jr. enjoyed the traditional liberal arts Yale College education. But he was also skilled in mechanical and scientific arts, which
were to be of great value in later life. He had not been exposed to a
training which would lead him into a life of pure research, a training
which for most individuals was then available only in Europe. His
temperament may have been such that he could never have been a pure
scientist. One writer who reviewed Ben's career commented, 'If he were
alive today, I like to think that he would be one of our leading chemical
Engineers.'[7]

Although both he and his father were well aware of the great advantages Europe had to offer and although Ben visited Europe twice for extended periods, he never enrolled in a European university of advanced study. With the exception of medical students, few Americans studied in Europe before the decade of the 1840s. Both Sillimans were soon advising their students that European study was essential if they were to be complete chemists, and it is clear that the younger Silliman regretted his lost opportunity. In 1854, he advised William Brewer, one of his students, as follows:

> I think that there is a glorious field in Physiological chemistry and my plan if I was of your age would be to go to Europe, perfect myself in general organic chemistry as a basis, study general and pathological anatomy at the same time and then turn in to the speciality of Physiological chemistry. What a work is that of Lehmann and . . . the Anatomical Chemistry of Robin and Verdeil! Such a preparation as I speak of would give a man great standing as a chemist and physiologist and open to him the best places in the country, which are in medical schools where such knowledge *made practical* and applied to the business of medicine, is most particularly wanted. This is what I should do if I were young again and had the same light I now have.[8]

Ben was able to keep abreast of European advances, since the *American Journal of Science,* of which he was an editor, received most of the important foreign publications as soon as they were available. In his capacity as editor and as an officer of various scientific societies, he soon either met every important scientist or corresponded with those he had not met. After graduation, the only formal training, other than that given by his father, seems to have been two months spent in the Boston laboratory of Dr. Charles T. Jackson in 1840.[9]

In 1837 Benjamin was appointed 'assistant to the professor of chemistry' at Yale, a title he held until 1840, when he was awarded the Master of Arts degree. Now Benjamin Silliman, Jr., A.M., he was confirmed as 'assistant in the Department of Chemistry, Mineralogy and Geology.' In 1842, the title of 'Lecturer' was added, and in 1846 he was appointed 'Professor of Chemistry and the Kindred Sciences as Applied to the Arts.' Unfortunately, these positions were poorly paid, and Benjamin, who enjoyed living well and whose family was growing, was forced to seek outside employment in order to augment his income (just as his father did).

In the first two years as assistant he was paid $357.46 and $415.24 respectively, sums which included board.[10] Some questions concerning these payments seem to have arisen, for the college Prudential Committee resolved in 1843 that the treasurer of the college ascertain on what authority the chemistry assistant was paid. Soon afterward, the Prudential Committee fixed his compensation at 'three Hundred Dollars a year for service in that department together with Seventy Dollars for Board.'[11] This was not to be the last inquiry made into the authority for paying Young Ben's compensation at Yale.

Because Ben lived at home before his marriage, he was at first able to live on this income, but since he continually purchased books, periodicals, and minerals, the need for money grew more intense. It should be noted that a Yale professor received $1,140 a year at this time. Tutors received $500. It was common knowledge that few faculty members could live on their salaries in the style that it was believed Yale professors should live. In 1850, a professor in the academic department was paid $1,300; $1,500 in 1854; $1,800 in 1856 and $3,000 in 1871.

In 1835, while still a junior at Yale, Ben assisted his father in a series of lectures at Salem, Massachusetts and Nantucket. 'Our son,' Benjamin Silliman remarked to his wife, 'is a great comfort and an important aid to me.'[12] Ben later helped his father with the Lowell Institute lecture series. For the 1842 series, Ben received $200 of the $2,000 taken in by his father.[13] Public lecturing had become very lucrative for Silliman by 1836. In 1835, for example, he collected more than $3,000 from lectures given in Salem, Boston, Lowell, Hartford, New Haven, Nantucket, and New York.[14] In 1845, the two Sillimans, father and son, embarked on a long lecture tour of the South. After expenses, and including receipts from lectures in Hartford and Brooklyn, they were left with $2,200, most of which probably went to the senior Silliman.[15] Benjamin Silliman, Jr. became an excellent popular lecturer and made a great deal of money from lectures in later years.

Ben emulated his father in inspecting steamboat and railroad locomotive boilers for insurance companies. He was usually required to travel to New York to carry on the steamboat inspections.

In 1835 Professor Silliman permitted townspeople to attend his geology lectures. So many New Haveners, particularly ladies, were attracted that students gave up their seats 'greatly to their inconvenience.'[16] By request he scheduled a special geology course for townspeople in which seventy men and women were enrolled. This lecture course was given an hour after his regular college lecture ended. In 1840 he turned these lectures over to Ben who gave twelve chemistry lectures in winter, followed by courses in mineralogy and geology. Ben had earlier given several lectures in chemistry to members of the Mechanics Institute in New Haven.

By 1840 Young Ben was also lecturing three times a week 'to a private class of students who desire to attend more particularly to mineralogy.'[17] In addition he was given the responsibility for teaching 'practical' science to those students who were interested, and in 1843, he taught two pupils privately in analytical chemistry.[18] The private laboratory teaching eventually evolved into the Sheffield Scientific School.[19]

Ben was especially busy during the college term because he was the major preparator for his father's lectures and to him fell the responsibility for maintaining the laboratory, ordering equipment and supplies, and keeping careful records and accounts. As early as 1838 he was deeply enmeshed in these duties. To Oliver P. Hubbard, a brother-in-law, and professor of chemistry, mineralogy, and geology at Dartmouth, Ben described the 'excellent . . . Berzelius' glasses' (beakers) in sizes from a half-pint to two quarts he had recently purchased in New York. These glasses were thin on the bottom in order to withstand heat, and could be nested. 'I need not tell you how useful they are . . . I think it would please you to see the apparatus room now in perfect order and as fast as time will permit I am going through the whole establishment in the same way.'[20]

During the first few years of Ben's assistantship, he was closely supervised by his father, especially so when they were preparing for a new lecture series. Even when he was away, Benjamin Silliman regularly wrote to remind his son of his duties. One letter lists seventeen separate chores such as 'I trust you have attended to the gazometer . . . The pneumatic cistern—the copper one . . . The seats cleaned. all apparatus and specimens both in laboratory and Cabinet in place . . . Office carpet up and shaken.'[21] Young Ben did not himself shake the office carpet, but he was at his father's command to see to it that all was ready. Benjamin Silliman, however, was always appreciative of his son's performance and commended him at every opportunity. 'My son,' he once wrote, 'has become a very able assistant and is zealous in action and studious in books so that he is fast advancing.'[22]

Ben soon began to perform the chemistry demonstrations for his father and even substituted for him in chemistry, mineralogy, and geology on those days when his father was away on business. In 1841 he lectured for a full week when Professor Silliman was called away to

Hartford and Boston. He was given a detailed outline leavened with good advice.[23]

> I would begin the preparations for each lecture in the afternoon as soon as you are through with a previous duty, and go over everything with your assistants so that you may all (and they in particular) acquire facility, that there may be no awkwardness.
>
> For the first lecture it may answer to begin to prepare on Monday morning,—but by no means [delay and avoid] any procrastination—spare time, if any, will come better after your mind is at ease as regards preparation. Remember, it is a capital opportunity to establish your reputation.

The elder Silliman soon became dependent on Young Ben. 'My son,' he noted in 1842, 'is my right hand and is growing more and more efficient and successful—but by absences in the cities (necessary and approved by me) and by illness, he has been away from the laboratory about half the course.'[24]

Even after the Department of Philosophy and the Arts and the Yale School of Applied Chemistry had begun to operate in 1847, and Ben took on heavy new responsibilities, he was required to help his father with the demonstrations, lectures, and recitations. Shortly after the new school began, Professor Silliman noted that 'I review one half of the Senior Class—BS Jr. the other.'[25]

In 1849 soon after Young Ben accepted a call to teach in the Medical Department of the University of Louisville in Kentucky, his father announced that he would resign his professorship, his resignation '. . . hastened by the loss of my son as assistant in the chemical department. The preparation and performance of very numerous chemical experiments before a collection of young men seems not to be very appropriate to a veteran who has passed his seventieth year.'[26]

Young Ben was often absent from his official duties. In 1845, for example, he was engaged by the Boston Water Board to analyze sources of drinking water for the growing city, and to recommend the best sources. When he returned from Boston after presenting his final report, he was 'highly gratified by the reception his report met with,' and by the fact that he was paid $500 for this work which was the first of a series of water studies he carried out during the next two decades for a number of cities.[27]

Ben was also engaged in analyzing the coral specimens brought back by James Dwight Dana from the Wilkes Expedition and was excused from helping his father in the geology course the spring of 1845.[28] Ben soon learned that the United States Congress was unwilling to pay him for these analyses. Dana had commissioned them 'with only a verbal permission from the judge [Senator Benjamin Tappan] which now, to my surprise, proves to be insufficient authority and there is doubt whether the bill will be paid.'[29] Ben convinced the Library Committee of Congress that he deserved compensation but received only $300 instead of the $600 which he had been promised, on the ground that his claim was irregular. He was forced to settle for this amount, although it was sufficient only to repay an advance Dana had given him from his own funds.[30]

On 15 April 1849, Young Ben was informed by Dr. Benjamin Yandell of the Medical Department of the University of Louisville that he would be offered 'an important and very lucrative post which has not been sought but has been spontaneously offered.'[31] The elder Silliman noted on at least two other occasions that his son's offer was 'entirely unsought' and 'unsolicited and unexpected.'[32]

Under the terms of his agreement with the Medical Department, Silliman, Jr. was obligated to teach in Louisville from November 1st to March 20th or 25th. Compensation would depend on fees and was estimated to be 'between 4 and 5 thousand dollars . . . for four months of labor.'[33] This was a tempting offer, although the level of compensation cited was never attained. Ben, who knew Louisville well, rented a house and moved his family there for several winters, returning to New Haven in the summer both to teach and to look after his other interests.

The appointment to the Louisville Medical Department was probably not as unsolicited as the elder Silliman insisted, since the Sillimans had many friends and former students in Louisville. They knew Dr. Yandell well and had visited the Medical Department at Louisville in 1845 as Yandell's guests.[34] Both surely had informed their many friends of Young Ben's excellent qualifications to serve as a professor in a medical school.

At Louisville, Ben was not content to confine himself to teaching. He fitted a private laboratory for students who wished to learn practical chemistry, although he was cautioned by his father about diversion of labor. 'It may be well,' the senior Silliman said, 'to have a few private pupils in analysis, but not many as they would interfere with your labors in the course to which everything else should yield.'[35]

During the first year or two in Louisville, Ben worked regularly in his laboratory: '[I] am as regular as a clock—rise at 7, breakfast 7 ½, Laboratory at 9, 1 ½ dine. Laboratory till 5. Sup at ¼ 6. Study and write until 12 or 1. Saturday night I usually retire earlier.'[36] But there were few students in the laboratory, and the pressure of his lecturing required a change in his routine.

> I am sorry to say that I have not done anything in work this winter. My experience is that five lectures a week and the numerous duties and cares of a professorship do not leave much time for research—But if I do not work myself, I like to have it go on about me and there has not been so much of that this winter as on some former occasion.[37]

The laboratory did not flourish. George Brush, Ben's assistant in 1851, noted that there was only one student at Louisville while he was there.[38] Brush wrote to tell his friend Brewer that if the laboratory became more popular, which was doubtful, Brewer could anticipate a position at Louisville. If he wished to come to study, 'the laboratory [will be] at your service as well as reagents . . . in addition, a hearty welcome from the managers.'[39]

Brush was pleased with the quality of Ben's laboratory, 'one of the nicest little rooms fitted up with 6 benches and plenty of little drawers (such as you and I like), a nice little cooking stove, sandbaths, etc.' There was a good quantity of supplies and equipment 'and lots of little nice things we did not have at the old [Yale] Analytical Laboratory. Tongs tipped with platinum and other *doings* of a similar nature.'[40]

The elder Silliman, who sorely missed his son, was delighted by Young Ben's success at Louisville:

> In my last I mentioned my satisfaction that you had gone through so well with your carbonic snow and frozen mercury and am much gratified by the very favorable notice by Dr. Yandell; it is very creditable both to you and him. I hope your other public lectures will go off as well and I think they will from the nature of the subjects. You will not forget the revolving flame of the magnet nor the galvanic light in vacuo; if your blowpipe experiments should need extension—the combustion of the metals will afford rich experiments—especially copper-lead-tin-bismuth and antimony; the latter dancing on the long wide board is you recollect very striking.[41]

Ben took Louisville by storm. When the medical doctors of the University of Louisville organized a Natural History Society, Ben was chosen to give the first of a series of public lectures beginning on 19 December 1851. These lectures were so popular that he finally gave six of the total of eight in 1851–52. Hundreds of people were turned away from the filled hall. Since Young Ben was a skilled demonstrator and a superlative lecturer, his audiences were enthralled by his demonstration of the oxyhydrogen blowpipe, the combustion of phosphorus in oxygen, and the art of taking daguerreotype pictures with the electric arc light. One knowledgeable listener noted 'the pleasure [Silliman] has given us by his public discourse during this and previous lectures.'[42]

The younger Silliman was regarded as 'the most popular lecturer of the faculty at Louisville.' Eliot Jarvis, who heard him at both Yale and Louisville, rather preferred him to his father. 'He gave a more complete view of his subject, and digressed but very little to tell stories, or mention "my friend, Dr. Hare."'[43] Jarvis, however, remarked that the class of '49 at Yale thought it 'very dull sport to hear "Young Ben."'

Not everyone in the West was enthusiastic about him, however, for Ben wrote his wife that:

> Some writer in the *Cincinnati Commercial* has attacked me in a very contemptuous style because of my letter to Guyot on Mammoth Cave—It has been copied in the Courier here, but I had the forbearance to burn the paper without reading the article and shall take no notice of it. I understand he tries to make fun of me and he says [?] that I have committed some terrible blunders. It has probably been written by some Dr. to injure the School here.[44]

Despite these popular successes, Silliman's income from the medical course was less than he had expected, $3,750 instead of $5,250. His class had enrolled only 250 students at fifteen dollars each instead of the 350 or more he had been told would attend.[45]

Ben seems to have deserved a reputation for enjoying a rather high life style and for spending, often in advance, money he made. There is no doubt that he was forced to live in a less opulent style as investment losses and his almost pathologically malicious enemies conspired to darken his life in later years. However, much of his income went to help his students, and to purchase mineral specimens, new books, and laboratory equipment.

> Neither luxurious nor penurious in his [Ben's] habits he saved a modest competence and for the rest spent liberally a handsome income, an income derived not from his chosen profession, for from the founding of the Yale scientific school he too often paid his own salary, and many an

earnest student can testify how freely his time, and means as well, have
been forced upon his pupils. There was the use he loved to make of the
dollars he received from the industries to which he had saved fortunes.[46]

This habit of spending liberally showed in the early years of his
marriage. Silliman, Jr. was fortunate in that he was never burdened by
the need to build his own house since William J. Forbes, his father-in-
law, built for his daughter and son-in-law a large home in Hillhouse
Avenue, only fifty yards away from Silliman, Sr.'s house. Benjamin
Silliman, Jr. and Susan Forbes were married in the spring of 1840 and
moved into the new house in May of that year, shortly after Mr. Forbes
died. The house, from which Ben was absent so much, was substantially remodeled from the proceeds of his extraordinary successes in
1864 as a mining and oil consultant in California. It was known as a
center of hospitality and friendship, since the Sillimans, father and
son, were so widely acquainted with distinguished men and women
who invariably visited the Sillimans when they were near New Haven.
'In the old days it [Silliman Jr.'s house] was always full of life and
gaiety and open hospitality and the four daughters who grew up there
were rarely lovely girls and greatly admired.'[47]

In 1851 he complained somewhat whimsically to his wife, who
remained in New Haven that winter while he taught at the Louisville
Medical School, about their excesses:

> How unlucky we are in our efforts at frugality! I estimate that in
> about two years and 3 or 4 months past we have received over thirteen
> thousand dollars and we are in debt now! I include in this $1000 from Mr.
> Norton for my laboratory rights in N.H. and I suppose I have probably at
> least that value on hand now of similar things—and I include also our
> earnings this winter of $3000 of which $2000 are now on hand and equal to
> our debts, but how are we to *live* and pay our debts. I suppose by going to
> Europe again . . . you are just as prudent and frugal as you can be I am
> sure and I think that we have both this winter been very saving for us. Two
> years of similar frugality will make us comfortable—It was one spending
> of $5000 in Europe which has eaten such a hole in our resources. But I
> trust we shall recover that bread cast on the waters also. Perhaps if we have
> two or three more children we shall be rich.[48]

Benjamin Silliman has often been honored for founding and
editing the *American Journal of Science*, which he carried on virtually
by himself at great personal sacrifice until his son began to help in

1838. In 1841 the name of Benjamin Silliman, Jr. joined that of Benjamin Silliman as editor, and remained on the masthead of the *American Journal of Science* until Ben's death in 1885. The addition of Young Ben as editor was to be expected since the elder Silliman loved his son, and believed strongly in his scientific ability. The father also delighted in the fact that Ben had become a good, if somewhat prolix writer, and soon relied as much on Ben's editorial services as on his laboratory assistance.

In 1847, in the preface to volume 50 of the *Journal*, Benjamin Silliman, in his 'Roman' manner referred to his son's service:

> On the title page of N. 1, vol. 34, published in July, 1838, a new name is introduced; the individual to whom it belongs having been for several years more or less concerned in the management of the Journal, and from his education, position, pursuits and taste, as well as from affinity, being almost identified with the editor, he seems to be quite a natural ally and his adoption into the editorship was scarcely a violation of individual unity. His assistance has proved to be very important;—his near relation to the senior editor prevents him from saying more, while justice does not permit him to say less.[49]

The addition of Benjamin to the editorial staff of the *American Journal of Science* did not meet with universal approbation from the community of scientists. Joseph Henry commented to Alexander D. Bache in 1838 about his complaints to Professor Silliman concerning some of the material in the *Journal*: 'He said if I could see what he rejected I would scarcely complain of what he inserted. I also hinted the importance of having colaborators [sic] in the different departments of science for a journal of this kind. The hint was not however taken and shortly after name of the Professors son was attached to the Journal.'[50]

This remark was probably occasioned more by the fact that Henry sought to 'raise . . . the scientific character' of American research than it was a criticism of Ben himself. Henry could obviously not accept a twenty-two year old youth barely out of college as the kind of important figure to edit the major American scientific publication. However, even though Ben lacked scientific prestige, he soon became indispensable to his father in both the financial and editorial aspects of publication.[51] His contributions as editor and writer were frequent and substantial. Alexander D. Bache was also cool to Ben's inclusion as a charter member of the National Academy of Sciences.[52]

The *Journal* was supported for many years by dint of prodigious personal effort and fund raising by the two Sillimans. On more than one occasion they borrowed substantial sums of money from Yale College to pay accumulated bills.[53] Their correspondence, especially when Ben was in Louisville, repeatedly refers to *Journal* topics, to bills to be paid, to contributors to reply to, to wood prints to be delivered, and to agents to be urged on ever more vigorously or, on occasion, to be changed. The several offers to sell the *Journal* were always refused.

Perhaps because both enjoyed living as they thought professors should live, a taste which forced them into extensive outside work, and because they were so deeply involved in the *American Journal of Science* with its steady stream of bills and receivables, the Sillimans carefully kept track of the monies owing and due each other:

> I have no doubt that the account is correct, although some items are new to me. I suppose that you received the Ray publications gratis from the Society as a compliment to yourself and had no idea of subscribing for the work. Have you any recollection of such an arrangement—I have not. . . . The Ray item in your debt to me is $40. The $23 . . . charged on account of transactions with Mr. Pease of this city—connected with some transaction with his brother I do not understand—but doubtless you do and can explain it, but as these things may be troublesome to discuss at such a distance of time and space it may be as well to preserve this note and let these matters rest until we meet again.[54]

By 1846, the year in which James Dwight Dana, Ben's brother-in-law, joined the editorial staff, the *Journal* was in a better financial position. Its circulation was approaching one thousand paid subscribers and the quality of the printed papers had improved. 'Our design,' Ben said, 'is to keep in advance of everybody.' He was optimistic that its influence in England seemed to have increased substantially since journals such as *Jameson's* printed large sections from the *Journal* 'and not always with acknowledgement of the source.'[55] Sales in England, however, had not increased markedly. Not more than seventy copies were sold in London.

In 1849, thirty-one years after the founding of the *Journal*, Benjamin Silliman, who had given much thought to its future, informed his son: 'As it now appears . . . that I have a very valuable property in the Journal I must have reference to it in my evening of life when property and other resources may fail.'[56]

In 1850 he decided to transfer ownership of the *Journal* to his son and to James Dwight Dana. The three drew up a formal agreement by which he retained title to all monies owed the *Journal* before 1 January 1851, to all numbers of the *Journal* published and on hand before that date, and to the copper plates, lithographic stones, wood cuts 'and other literary property' prior to volume 1 of the second series which had begun with the January 1846 issue. In addition his name was to remain on the cover as senior editor, and he would 'generally [do] all in his power to promote the interests of the work.'

The younger Silliman and Dana agreed to serve as agents for the sale of back issues, to receive for these services a commission of 25% on all sales made after 1 January 1851. In addition they agree to pay Professor Silliman $300 a year from net proceeds. If the net exceeded $1,000, he was to receive 25% of the excess. The two young editors could charge up to $300 a year for editorship and $200 for clerkship against income. They were also allowed to keep all publications sent in exchange except those sent expressly as gifts to the senior editor.[57] When the elder Silliman died in 1864, he left an estimated $1,000 worth of back numbers of the *Journal* to the two editors.[58] In 1878, Ben, characteristically in need of money, sold his half-interest in the *Journal* for $1,500 to Dana. He continued to be listed on the cover as 'one of the 2 editors-in-chief' and was to continue with 'such editorial duties as he may be able to perform without further compensation,' as well as keep 'such serials as have heretofore come to his share in the regular course of exchange.'[59]

There is good reason to believe that Professor Silliman sought to persuade the Yale Corporation to appoint Ben as his successor after his first resignation in 1849. Toward the end of 1849 he wrote Ben: 'Nothing transpires here regarding my successor—but I will not say anything more of that topic now, perhaps I may even write to you a separate confidential note on that important affair—waive it for the present.'[60] Several months later Ben informed Dr. Yandell that his father was becoming more cheerful: 'The natural elasticity of his mind has returned since he decided to retain his place in College and that great source of trial has been removed—the feeling that his views and opinions regarding his successor were held of light regard.'[61] As late as January 1853, Ben was not convinced that he would succeed his father at Yale. 'We are ¾ through here [Louisville] for this season, now my fourth in Louisville ... possibly it may be my last—but as our foresight is never (as the Dutchman said) so good as our hindsight it will be easier to predict what will happen when we know.'[62]

There seems to have been considerable opposition in New Haven to Ben's appointment. Mason Weld, one of his students who had also assisted the elder Silliman, wrote to Ben in 1854 to seek advice on a future career, and to apologize for remarks he was reported to have made when Ben's appointment was in doubt.

> It is true that there were many reports floating in regard to yourself that had a certain degree of plausibility—and this was just at the time when there was doubt thrown, and this in the minds of some persons unacquainted with the true state of the case, on the probability of your succeeding your father, and I was enquired of by multitudes of curious and interested persons, and drawn in conversation to speak of things of which I happily knew nothing or next to nothing because people thought that I must know or be able to judge. I might have said injudicious things or things which you might think were prejudicial to your interests but I do not think I did, for at this time I was regarding your return to New Haven permanently as the only proper arrangement and was feeling the need of your presence in N.H. very much—In the laboratory, the students, assistants and all were working, following books and each other, without any practical teacher, one who worked with us, or could show us how to work by ourselves. We would have prized ½ hour a week from anyone who knew and would have given hints, answered questions or offered explanations—this, you will remember was at the time of Prof. Norton's sickness or when he was so much engaged with lecturing in Albany and New Haven.[63]

In February 1853 President Woolsey wrote to Benjamin Silliman, Sr. to inform him that the Prudential Committee would nominate Benjamin Silliman, Jr. to give the college and medical school lectures in chemistry during the first term, and that 'part of these instructions ought to be from textbooks.' In addition, since Ben was already a professor in the Department of Philosophy and the Arts, he would not be required to participate in the college government. The salary was to be $1,000, the college to bear laboratory costs, or $1,300 if he would bear the costs. In addition, there would be reduced funding for assistants.[64]

This must have wounded the venerable teacher severely. Although Benjamin would be ranked as a professor at Yale College, he would not be a member of the Academical Faculty, which was the heart of the institution, and was specifically excluded from its governance. Certainly this professorship was less prestigious than that which James Dwight Dana held. A decade later, after the Peabody endowment had been announced, O. C. Marsh, then seeking Ben's recommendation for a Yale professorship, was afraid that Ben lacked influence with the Yale

Corporation because 'he is only a Professor in the Medical Department.' [65] Despite this, Marsh was confident a few months later that he would be appointed professor of geology and palaeontology as soon as he had properly prepared himself because of an assurance to this effect from both Dana and Ben, 'with whom the appointment rests.' [66] There may have been some difference in status—there certainly was in salary, but it is clear that Ben and, of course, Benjamin Silliman, Sr., were not without influence of their own.

Once the recommendation of the Prudential Committee had been made, it was certain that Benjamin Silliman, Jr. would be appointed to another professorship at Yale.

Ben, however, seems to have been of two minds about leaving his post in Louisville. Although his father noted Ben's 'mental conflict in coming to a decision of the great question,' the elder Silliman never questioned the inevitability of the decision; and he was direct in discussing the matter and manner of compensation, how fees were to be arranged and how much Ben would be permitted to keep. He informed Ben that President Woolsey had voluntarily agreed to continue the $100-a-year expense allowance for supplies from the medical school; that he could retain half the fees of the townfolk who attended his lectures; and that he would be given some paid laboratory assistance. [67] Shortly before he left Louisville, the younger Silliman complained that since his classes at Louisville were larger than before, and now some 300 students, he was making 'a very large pecuniary sacrifice in leaving it.' [68]

There was also some discussion about the scientific school at Yale which was in disorder after John Pitkin Norton's death. The elder Silliman seemed to think there would be a good opportunity for Ben to move into a position of leadership, and, together with John A. Porter (who had been proposed as the next professor of analytical and agricultural chemistry and was then acting director of the school), to divide the income of the school equitably. [69] This scheme was never implemented. In 1854, when it seemed likely that Porter would leave Yale for Columbia College, the elder Silliman looked forward to the possibility that his son would direct the scientific school at Yale. Together, Silliman thought, he and his son could raise enough money to put the scientific school on a firm financial footing. 'In the end,' he said, 'you may find it a source of emolument to you and perhaps could conduct it alone with the aid of your pupils.' [70]

After Professor Silliman's resignation was finally accepted by the Yale Corporation on 26 July 1853, the corporation resolved:

That Prof. B. Silliman, Jun. be appointed to take the place in the Medical Department made vacant by the resignation of his father.

Prof. Silliman, Jun. be requested to take charge of the instruction in chemistry in the academic department.

. . . that B. Silliman, Jun. Professor in the Medical and Philosophical Departments be requested to take charge of the instruction in Chemistry in the Acad. Department and that his compensation for this service be for the present $1000 dollars without expenses, or 1300 dollars (he defraying the expenses of the Laboratory) as he shall elect.[71]

Ben's statement of his reasons for leaving Louisville, given to the graduating medical class of 1854, was eloquently phrased:

The last accents of the present occasion close my relationship with this institution. Fain would I hold the cadence, but I must forbear. We act wisely in this world when we follow the leadings of Providence and I seem to discern not unequivocally that the indications of a controlling destiny call me to other duties in a distant state. I will not detain you to recount the strife of equally balanced or of contrasting interests, feelings, duties [by] which I have reached the conclusion which decides my action.[72]

In 1855 Benjamin's compensation was increased to $1,400, an amount $100 more than he was paid the previous year.[73] In 1856 it was increased to $1,500. The salary of a professor in the academical department was $1,800 at that time.

Ben, who well knew the condition of the Yale laboratory, gave a great deal of thought to its needs and discussed with his father certain improvements which he thought should be made. His father was in complete agreement.

I think that all you propose as to additional means to refit the laboratory is unassailable and I will give my influence to have it carried. I still have a vote in both faculties. Robert [his faithful assistant] says that there has never been such havoc in the Laboratory. Young P. and an Irishman . . . a good chemist, but careless and heavy handed, have demolished most of the glass. Now will be a good time to put in for a new laboratory, as it is quite time—but much will depend upon the success of the subscription.[74]

In a letter addressed to the president and fellows of Yale College, Ben described the run-down state of the laboratory, and proposed 'to supply these deficiencies in a systematic and permanent manner with the view of establishing a museum and collection of chemical apparatus' when sufficient funds were available. For the 1854–55 year, he requested $600 for 'our most urgent wants.' Since the present laboratory was in a 'very dilapidated condition, so badly adapted for its objects, having been designed for a wholly different purpose,' a new building would be needed.[75]

Six hundred dollars was voted by the corporation, but Ben imprudently overspent this appropriation by more than $500. This action led to an investigation by the Prudential Committee of the college which was authorized by the corporation to examine Ben's accounts to determine if the additional payment was justified. The Prudential Committee, following an extended discussion on 27 July 1855, voted the money 'with the understanding distinctly stated that hereafter no bills for chemical apparatus or supplies will be allowed beyond the appropriations.'[76]

Although Silliman, Jr.'s title on his appointment to the Department of Philosophy and the Arts had variously been given as 'Professor of Applied Chemistry' and 'Professor of Chemistry and the Kindred Sciences as applied to the Arts,' the corporation affirmed on 28 July 1857 that his title was 'to be, as now, Professor of General and Applied Chemistry.' In 1872 it was changed without explanation to 'Professor of Chemistry.'

Benjamin Silliman, Jr. was a prolific writer. The number of articles, research reports, book reviews, and notes by him in the *American Journal of Science* and in other periodicals, signed and unsigned, is prodigious. In addition to periodical literatures, he edited or himself wrote a number of books, monographs, and pamphlets. His first effort in this direction was the preparation of an American edition of Liebig's *Organic Chemistry in Its Applications to Agriculture and Physiology* which, however, he withdrew before its publication when he learned that Professor Webster at Harvard was seeing an edition of this work through the press.[77] His second was an American edition of Gerardus Mulder's *The Chemistry of Vegetable and Animal Physiology* which appeared in 1845 with little notice from the public.

Ben soon turned to the preparation of a chemistry textbook for schools and colleges. He was not the only Yale faculty member who wrote textbooks since a number of professors had already produced successful textbooks, which enabled them to increase substantially their college salary of a little more than a thousand dollars. The market for textbooks in the United States was large and growing rapidly. In the fifty years between 1820 and 1870, more than 200 chemistry texts alone were published in the United States, ranging from books for beginners to advanced texts. By 1853, Mrs. Marcet's *Conversations* had sold over 160,000 copies, and Youman's *Classbook of Chemistry*, first published in 1860, had sold more than 140,000 copies.[78]

His *First Principles of Chemistry* appeared in 1847, and Ben was soon pleased to receive $300 for the 3,000 copies sold early that year.[79] The third edition, published in 1852, fifty years after Benjamin Silliman, Sr. was appointed professor of chemistry and natural history at Yale, was dedicated as follows: 'To Benjamin Silliman, for Fifty years Professor of Chemistry in Yale College, This Volume, designed to promote that science, to which he has devoted his life, is respectfully dedicated by his son.' Although it was far behind George Fownes *Manual of Elementary Chemistry*, an English textbook, Ben's text which appeared in three major editions was widely used, and was especially popular in medical schools. It was one of the most frequently adopted American medical school texts of the fifties and sixties.[80] In 1850 in the academies of New York State it was second only to Comstock's *Chemistry*, having been adopted by some thirty schools; and as late as 1880 it was still used by many normal schools as a reference text, having been superseded as a primary text by the phenomenally successful chemistry books written by Joel Dorman Steele and E. L. Youmans.

The *First Principles of Chemistry* is notable for clear and succinct explanations, and also for a major section on organic chemistry. This section was written and revised in each edition by T. Sterry Hunt, Ben's assistant in his private analytical laboratory in the early 1840s. Although Hunt was not granted coauthorship as one might have expected from the extent of his contribution, a third of the total work, Ben continued 'to acknowledge his obligations to his friend and former associate, Mr. Hunt, for his lucid and original exposition of this part of the subject.'[81] Hunt, however, was probably well paid for his contribution, especially as his own reputation as a scientist grew.

Benjamin Silliman, Jr., like so many past and present authors, tried to promote his book. In 1853, shortly after the third edition of his textbook had appeared, Ben asked, after remarking that Brewer should already have received a copy from the publisher, 'Can you not send me a list of names of teachers in N.Y. to whom it would be worthwhile to send copies of the book?'[82]

One of its major strengths, aside from the intrinsically good qualities of the book, was that its author was professor of chemistry at Yale, and his textbook was naturally used at Yale. From the beginning of his teaching career at Yale in the School of Applied Chemistry, Ben required that his book be used. When he was called to his new duties at Yale in 1854, he immediately required his textbook for the scientific, the academical, and the medical school students. He supplemented it and his lectures with two editions of a chemistry syllabus based on the book.

In 1858 he published a physics textbook for use in academies and colleges. Although not as popular as his chemistry, especially in the academies and high schools, it was used for years in many colleges, and went through a second edition and several revisions. Ben once again turned to his friends to seek suggestions for improvement. In 1859 he wrote Brewer to say: 'I shall be very happy to receive your suggestions and criticisms for a new edition which I am now working at and hope to have out in 2 mos.'

He was also planning a major revision of his chemistry book and in 1859 wrote to Brewer, 'The Chemistry I mean to make a compound of the excellences of Fourier, Stockhardt and my own book. If the mixture is adroitly made I shall be able to concoct a better book for students than now exists.'[83] A month later, he thanked Brewer for his 'valuable suggestions respecting .the Philosophy—they were most timely and I trust you will run through the other chapters in the same way. . . . All your suggestions will receive mature consideration.'[84] There is no acknowledgment of Brewer's contributions, however, in the second edition of the physics book, which was substantially improved. This edition is noteworthy in that it was one of the first American textbooks to incorporate problems and solutions based on scientific principles. The text was reorganized into chapters, and the practice problems were placed at the end of each chapter. 'Those who know how to do so,' he said, 'will use them while others will pass them.'[85]

These books written to present difficult concepts to scientifically unsophisticated students were exemplary teaching instruments. Although they were formidably bulky, they contained a minimum of advanced mathematics. There was an abundance of instructive wood cuts, and the important scientific principles were illustrated in their practical applications. Young Ben was masterful in elucidating such relationships. He had, as one recent writer has commented, a 'remarkable ability to synthesize, explain, and extract from the work of others with great clarity and effectiveness.'[86]

Ben was popular with his students, although there seemed to be some feeling that he 'is conscious of himself and all he does.' This comment was made by a student who allowed, however, that Silliman, Jr. was 'goodnatured and worthy of esteem.'[87] Norton, on the other hand, 'seemed lost in the effort to please and be useful to others. We studied and taught agr. chem. because he lived it, as his science; and he seemed to possess a warm, personal interest in all who had a taste for similar pursuits.'[88] Not all of Norton's students, however, shared this favorable view.

In later years, F. B. Dexter commented that Ben 'lectured in such a flowery style that his attainments seemed "brilliant rather than solid."'[89] Dexter also criticized other well-known Yale faculty members for poor teaching. Ben seems to have modeled his lecturing on his father's style, and, as his lecture notes indicate, he became more prolix as he grew older. His father had early cautioned him to avoid excess: 'You will no doubt prepare thoroughly and execute with tact and uniform success—and give luminous and condensed explanations and do not indulge in digression or sportiveness except sparingly.'[90] The elder Silliman was a notably discursive lecturer, and it is probable that he was warning his son to avoid complete emulation.

Ben's students thought he was not only an excellent lecturer but also 'one of the finest gentlemen in existence.'[91] Ben enjoyed his students and sought to help them whenever possible. He wrote letters of reference for them untiringly, and vigorously sought suitable positions for them, positions which were difficult to find. George Brush once wrote to W. H. Brewer that Ben had referred to him as follows: 'A noble fellow is Brewer and I [Ben] wish him well from the bottom of my heart.' Brush added that, 'He [Ben] will always be ready to aid you and when you want a good word you will have it from him.'[92] Brush was overwhelmed when Ben wrote to Brush's father to seek permission for Brush to accompany Ben and his father on their trip to Europe. 'Was it not kind in young Ben to write to the old gentleman. Oh! I wish you were to go with us. Could not *we* have a good time.'[93]

Ben frequently intervened for his students, gave his advice freely, and lent them money ($500 to Brewer, which was somewhat grudgingly repaid). There may well have been some Freudian compensation on Brewer's part, stemming from his early reliance on Young Ben, when some years later Brewer turned against his former teacher and became one of his most vigorous enemies, even attempting to force Ben to resign from Yale.[94] When Ben was appointed to direct the Department of Chemistry and Mineralogy at the Crystal Palace Exhibition of 1854 at New York City, he employed several of his students as assistants, and saw to it that they were mentioned in the publications he edited.

Ben's interest in his students continued throughout his life. In 1858, he wrote Brewer who was soon to desert him:

I wish you had a professorship worthy of your talents and ability to teach. . . . Such a good fellow as you are ought not to be losing the flower of your youth but should have it nicely tied up on a love knot and I hope you may be nightly visited by pleasant visions of an angel bearing a white lily in his hand, your sweet annunciation, of a real joy in store for you.[95]

In 1863 Ben told Brewer about a possible bounty, under the Agricultural College Bill, of 200,000 acres of land, which might be turned into enough money to establish a chair at Yale for Brewer to fill. He also suggested that if George Brush were forced to return to New Haven, Brush might work at the laboratory and live in an apartment in the Sheffield School, 'a large unoccupied room intended as a museum.'[96]

One remarkable aspect of this interest in his students (which less kindly critics might call student exploitation) was Ben's habit of depending on students for analytical work often carried out with a minimum of supervision. Such dependence caused him considerable embarrassment on more than one occasion. Nevertheless, Ben scrupulously gave the students credit for assistance, no matter how minute, thus bringing them to international attention. Most of his research was first published in the *American Journal of Science*, which was circulated throughout the civilized world and portions of which were often reprinted in European journals.

T. Sterry Hunt and John Pitkin Norton, probably Ben's best known students, came from his private analytical laboratory in the early 1840s. Hunt, who became one of America's most eminent chemists and geologists, published more than 400 papers on chemical and geological topics and never wavered in his loyalty to Ben. Hunt worked with Ben in 1845 and 1846, and showed remarkable ability. George P. Merrill was somewhat critical of Hunt's general influence on American geology but called him an 'exceptionally brilliant man' and a 'versatile and brilliant genius.'[97] Hunt's only formal scientific training was the two years in New Haven. Yet by February 1847, at the age of twenty-one, Hunt left to take a post as chemist and mineralogist to the Geological Survey of Canada, having been appointed in August of 1846, a year and a half after coming to New Haven. By then he had already published eighteen articles and notes in the *American Journal of Science.*

In 1848 Hunt returned to New Haven to visit his old friends and stayed at 34 Hillhouse Avenue, Ben's home. Benjamin Silliman noted in his Day Book that 'Hunt was instructed here a friendless youth and by well doing has through our influence obtained this honorable appointment with a salary of $1200 per ann.'[98] In 1885 in a memorial tribute to his 'old friend and master,' Hunt referred to the years with Young Ben:

> The history of the work carried on by Silliman in the two years which I passed in that laboratory is instructive. Then and there were examined many of the materials brought home by the Wilkes Exploring Expedition, and the ores from Lake Superior and from Mine La Motte in Missouri, besides which a series of studies of potable waters was undertaken for the city of Boston.[99]

Ben always gave Hunt full credit for his work. In the preface to the first edition of his chemistry textbook, he presciently remarked:

> The organic chemistry is presented mainly in the order of Liebig in his *Traité de Chimie Organique*. The author takes pleasure in acknowledging the important aid derived in this portion of the work from his friend and professional assistant, Mr. Thomas S. Hunt, whose familiarity with the philosophy and details of Chemistry will not fail to make him one of its ablest followers. The labor of compiling the Organic Chemistry has fallen almost solely upon him.[100]

In papers written during the years when he was instructing laboratory students, Silliman, Jr. thanked George Weyman, Henri Erni, Denison Olmsted, Jr., William Craw, Joseph Crooke, Ludwig Stadtmuller, George Brush, Charles H. Rockwell and B. W. Bull, all students, for their contributions.[101]

At the meeting of the American Association for the Advancement of Science held in New Haven in 1850, William Craw, then the first assistant in the analytical laboratory, read a paper entitled 'Analysis of Phlogopite Micas from St. Lawrence County, New York.' A lively discussion followed among the distinguished scientists present in which Craw's method of determining fluorine was criticized. Ben came quickly to Craw's defense—he had probably suggested the topic and method to Craw in the first place—and commented that Craw's research confirmed his own optical examinations of these mica specimens. He added that 'Mr. Craw's paper must be regarded as one of much interest' because it would help mineralogists to separate phlogopites and muscovites.[102]

Throughout his productive lifetime, Silliman, Jr. engaged actively in a bewildering variety of industrial mining, lecturing, consulting, and teaching affairs, interests which kept him busy. He was a founder and director of the New Haven Gas Light Company, an early industrial interest which continued until his death. Baltimore, in 1816, was the first city in the United States to introduce gaslighting, and a number of other cities soon built gaslighting systems. In 1847 New Haven was the smallest city yet to plan such a system. With other New Haveners, mainly businessmen and bankers, Ben petitioned the legislature on 3 May 1847 for a charter to form a gas company. The petition became effective on 14 June 1847 when the New Haven Gas Light Co. formally came into being.[103]

Henry Hotchkiss Townsend, a member of an old New Haven family, commented that 'professor Benjamin Silliman, Jr. keenly alive as he always was to everything new, became actively interested in lighting by gas as a vast improvement over the methods New Haven then used.'[104] The nine incorporators raised $100,000 locally to build a gas plant and to lay four miles of gas mains from the gas plant in the eastern section of the city to its center. The first private home to be illuminated by gas was Ben's own which brightened the Thanksgiving Eve of 1848. The company prospered, and by 1856 it had more than 1,220 customers. As early as 1850, it had begun to pay a 6% dividend.[105] Ben held twenty shares of stock (which he was probably given without cost for his name and services) of the total of 4,000 shares.[106] He served actively on the Board of Directors, usually on the Distribution and Finance Committees. The Distribution Committee was responsible for locating the gas mains throughout the city. He also headed the Works Committee which supervised daily operations, recommended improvements in the plant, and supervised the construction of new facilities. Although he could not attend every meeting of the board since he was away from New Haven so much (some years he missed all or nearly all of the meetings) Benjamin Silliman, Jr.'s attendance record when he was in New Haven was excellent. Beginning in 1857, when he published 'Notice of a photometer and of some experiments therewith upon the comparative Power of Several Artificial Means of Illuminations' in the *Journal*, Silliman, Jr. carried on an active research program in gaslighting and frequently published on this topic, in this country and in England.

In 1853, Benjamin Silliman, Jr. was commissioned by the Association for the Exhibition of the Industry of All Nations to take charge of 'Mining, Mineralogical and Chemical Departments' for a major exhibition in the New York City Crystal Palace to be held in 1854. In order to develop these exhibits properly, he not only employed some of his former students, but also commissioned James Dwight Dana, Oliver Payson Hubbard, Dr. F. A. Genth, James Hall, David A. Wells, and

Charles Wetherill to scour the mining industry for appropriate exhibits, and to write appropriate commentaries.[107] This part of the exhibition must have been a prodigious labor since it included 287 mineral and mining exhibits from the United States, Nova Scotia, England, Ireland, Scotland, Wales, New Brunswick, and continental Europe. Of the 159 chemical and pharmaceutical exhibits, only 56 came from the United States—the majority were brought from Europe.[108] Ben's own collection of minerals, including native copper and silver from the Lake Superior mines and more than 150 specimens 'illustrating some of the best known or most noted localities and species' must have been one of the highlights.[109]

Soon after the exhibition opened, Ben furthered his career as a mining consultant when he served as one of three appraisers appointed by the governor of the state of Kentucky to investigate the Breckenridge Cannel Coal Company property.[110] Ben was an experienced coal mine and iron ore appraiser. As early as 1838 he and his father had been employed by the Maryland and New York Coal and Iron Company to visit a mine near Frostburgh, Maryland and to report on its commercial possibilities. In addition to examining its topographical and geological features, they collected a large number of coal and iron ore samples which they analyzed with the assistance of Charles U. Shepard. Their report, jointly signed, was optimistic, and one which would please the proprietors. However, the English owners were not content and called in other experts, including a mining engineer from England, who supported the Sillimans' conclusions. Coal and iron ore samples were also sent to England and analyzed by David Mushet and Andrew Ure, among others, who pronounced them of excellent quality and confirmed the analyses made by the Yale chemists.[111] At about this time, Ben met Charles W. Wheatley, the owner of the Wheatley Silver Lead Mines at Phoenixville, Pennsylvania, and formed a friendship with him that continued for many years. In 1864, when he sold certain holdings in these mines, Ben received some $130,000. He cheered up his wife, who was depressed because he was away so much, with the exclamation that '[I] was never in sight of so much money in my life.'[112]

In 1855 Benjamin Silliman, Jr. was president of the Connecticut Steam Heating Company. He remained connected with this firm, through several reorganizations, for more than twenty years. His zealous and certainly, in this case, questionable mode of operation, led him to write, in an advertising pamphlet, a short essay explaining the scientific and technical principles of his company's steam heating system. He signed this report 'Benjamin Silliman, Jr., Professor of General and Applied Chemistry in Yale College.' The pamphlet also included a letter from Silliman addressed to the secretary of the company about the steam heating system which had been installed in his own home. Ben reported favorably, stating that it was 'very much to my satisfaction and that of my family.'[113] Although a man of science, in this advertising testimonial, Young Ben revealed himself as an unscientific huckster:

> Experience will no doubt suggest improvements in this as in every new system, but we are confident that such improvements are to be looked for much more in the modifications of form in the apparatus and in the applications of good taste in decoration, than in any change of principle, which we believe to be now nearly perfect.[114]

Denison Olmsted, professor of natural philosophy, also a member of the board of the company, did not write such a testimonial.

Subsequent versions of this pamphlet, issued as late as 1875, included Silliman, Jr.'s essay on the principles of steam heating almost verbatim. The company seems to have prospered, and the list of satisfied customers throughout the country printed in each edition was long. In his capacity as scientific adviser to his company, Ben appeared before a committee of the New York City Board of Education to testify to the merits of the steam heating system manufactured by the American Automatic Steam Heating Company, an affiliate of his company, which was seeking adoption of its heating system by the New York public schools.[115] In 1866, while visiting Cleveland, he happily reported to Susan: '*Our* system of steam heating is very much in use here. Mr. Goodrich has it. This hotel is warmed exclusively by it and so are a large number of private and public buildings.'[116]

The variety of business projects described above is but a sampling from his incredibly busy career. Ben was a popular member of the New Haven Common Council from 1845 to 1849, receiving the largest number of votes of any candidate for office in the city election of 1848. The relationships established then were useful in founding and operating the New Haven Gas Light Company; cooperation from city authorities was surely necessary if the company were to prosper.

Ben was strongly interested in scientific agriculture during the decade of the 1840s, but turned from his pioneering role in it when he left New Haven in 1849. His course of eight lectures on agricultural chemistry given in New Orleans in 1845 upon the invitation of leading commercial and professional men there was the 'first course of lectures on that subject given in the United States.'[117] Ben was prepared for this task since he was an enthusiastic advocate of Justus Liebig and J. W. F. Johnston (perhaps too enthusiastic) and was well acquainted with what the leading theoreticians had to say about chemistry applied to agriculture.[118] He and his father were active members of the New Haven Horticultural Society and had some opportunity to become acquainted with the more practical aspects of agriculture. Young Silliman was an officer of this society and of the County Agricultural Society. In addition he, or perhaps more accurately, his gardener, often won prizes for fruit and vegetables grown in his garden.

In 1843 Ben, who had been active in the Association of American Geologists and Naturalists for several years, was elected secretary. He prepared the report of the 1843 meeting for publication in the *American Journal of Science*, and, perhaps because of his role with the *Journal*, the two Sillimans, together with Dana, planned the 1845 association meeting in New Haven.[119] The famous 'Rock Oil' study of 1855 was Benjamin's most important piece of geological research.[120] It provides insight into Ben's scientific ability and his business acumen. For example, it has been suggested that Ben was influenced by his heavy interest in the New Haven Gas Light Company to minimize the potential of petroleum in the production of illuminating gas.[121]

Ben continued to serve as a mining consultant. In 1854 he and James Hall visited a coal field in the Big Sandy River region of eastern Kentucky in which there was a possibility of their financial involvement. They withdrew from a syndicate formed to exploit this coal field because of a 'serious moral dereliction' by the leader of the syndicate. In this case Ben 'showed a sensitivity he lost later on.' He told the geologist J. P. Lesley that 'a man of science loses caste by having his name connected with anything of this sort in a public way.' Earlier he had confided to Lesley that a successful speculation could provide both Hall and himself 'plenty of sea room . . . for pure science (thereafter).'[122]

From the perspective of 120 years, one of Benjamin Silliman, Jr.'s most interesting entanglements was as manager of the Bristol Copper Mine in Bristol, Connecticut. This mine, in existence for years before his involvement (his father had surveyed it in 1839) was a profitable operation. Ben knew the mine well since he had often taken his students on field trips there. They were welcomed by Ludwig Stadtmuller, a former student, who was the operating manager at that time. In 1855 Ben and Josiah D. Whitney, who, in ten years became his most implacable enemy, jointly wrote a short, enthusiastic report on the mine at the invitation of Dr. Eliphalet Nott, president of Union College.[123] Nott controlled the mine. Their report was so favorable that Nott bought out the other owners, and organized a new company of which he was president and majority stockholder. Ben and Whitney were given some shares as partial compensation for their work, and with good reason. Their report was a mine owner's dream. 'By a judicious and moderate outlay, it can be made to return the whole cost of its plant and extraordinary expenses, with a wide margin of profit to the venture. . . . It is our conviction that the hope of future discoveries of great value in the continued exploration of the mine, was never more allied to certainty in any similar enterprise.'[124] The younger Silliman was soon named president of the mining company. John M. Woolsey, son of Theodore D. Woolsey, Yale President from 1846–1871, also had stock and was said to be an 'expert advisor.'[125]

There is a strong likelihood that the results of this venture contributed significantly to the success of Ben's enemies, including J. D. Whitney, his former partner, in making life at Yale so difficult for Ben in the late sixties and seventies. The Bristol Copper Mine venture was viewed with some apprehension by his brother-in-law, James Dwight Dana, who wrote to George Brush that 'B. S. Jr. is on the constant go in behalf of one thing or another, and alas for Science . . .'[126] But Ben needed money to take care of his growing family, and science was forced to take a back seat. The mine prospered for a short time under the new managers, and 'ore of exceeding richness was taken out in vast quantities.' Soon, however, expense exceeded income and Nott sold out. Then, 'under the direction of Prof. Silliman, the most extravagant schemes and experiments, of a costly nature were indulged in, the Professor being a fine theorist, but a very poor practical miner.'[127] In 1857 the Bristol Mining Company, whose prospects were so bright in 1855, went bankrupt.

Management extravagance was not the only cause; a financial recession was partially responsible. The mine itself was beset with a major problem: the copper veins were not continuous and bodies of copper ore were embedded in masses of barren rock.[128] Some expensive mechanical contrivances planned by Young Ben and built expressly for the mine, namely, a copper separator and a smelting furnace built to burn wet peat, failed to work effectively.[129] One writer commented that: 'Silliman infused all the enthusiastic energy and impractical methods of the theoretical scientist into the working details of the mine. Money was poured like water into the hole in the ground and was dissipated like clouds before the gale. Scheme after scheme was tried on the most extravagant scale. . . .'[130] Ben denied the charge of poor management in a letter not published until 1889: 'A letter from Prof. Silliman in Colorado, who was a large share-holder in the mine a year before it was abandoned, states that the mine was paying well but he became aware that the extravagant management would bring disastrous results and therefore he disposed of his interests a year before business was suspended.'[131]

This statement conflicts with Ben's sworn statement in the Moses Thompson 'Wet Fuel Furnace' case in 1871 when he testified that in May or June of 1857 he was 'engaged in mining explorations' at the Bristol mine and had ordered the Thompson furnaces which burned wet peat to be built. 'Thompson,' he said, 'proceeded to erect for the company which I then represented a block of four of his furnaces.'[132] Ben also stated that in 1857 he was president of the company.[133] If the newspaper quotations were correct, then it is clear that Silliman was attempting to escape responsibility for the mine failure by a patently untrue statement.

In 1855, the busy year in which he wrote the famous 'Rock Oil' report and became deeply involved with the Bristol mine, Benjamin wrote a favorable report on the marble quarry in Falls Village, Connecticut. 'Your quarry,' he said, 'will furnish, at the least, as good a material as any American marble now in use. . . . More than this you need not ask.'[134] The owner, F. R. Slocum, circulated a flyer which featured Ben's recommendation of his marble signed 'Professor of General and Applied Chemistry in Yale College.'

In April 1855 the two Sillimans spent two exhausting weeks looking into a copper vein in the Blue Ridge Mountains of Virginia. The elder Silliman was then seventy-five years old, and it was the last time he served as a mining consultant. In December 1855 Ben completed a report on the Williston Mine in Southampton, Massachusetts at the request of William Duryea, president of this New Haven–owned company. Although optimistic about the amount and quality of galena in the large quartz veins, Silliman, Jr.'s report is quite moderate and conservative. Ben recommended improvements such as a twenty or thirty horsepower steam engine and crusher like the one then in use at his Bristol Copper Mine.

All this time Ben was still teaching chemistry to Scientific School students, medical students, and to college seniors. He had also turned to the needs of his department and of the Scientific School for additional funding. He had earlier shown his ability as a fund raiser when, in 1843, he raised $2,200 from private sources to purchase for Yale the mineral cabinet of Baron Lederer, the Austrian consul-general in the United States. The Yale Corporation contributed an additional $600 for the project and paid the expenses Ben incurred in the course of his campaign.[135] The same year he persuaded Nathan Appleton, a Boston industrialist, to give $500 to support publication of the *Proceedings of the Association of American Geologists and Naturalists* of which Ben served as one of the editors.[136]

In 1854 Silliman, Jr. was appointed by the Prudential Committee of Yale College as an agent in 'raising funds for the College, his compensation to be 5 percent on monies obtained by him for the corporation.'[137] There is no indication of his success in this task, however. Some years earlier, when Ben was corresponding with John Pitkin Norton, then studying at Mulder's laboratory in Utrecht, Holland, he offered to raise $20,000 which could be 'obtained immediately and without any difficulty.'[138] Unfortunately, Ben was much too optimistic and nothing approaching this sum was raised during Norton's lifetime.

In 1856 a new campaign to raise funds for the Scientific School was launched. The amount needed was set at $150,000. Ben and Dana were the committee of professors who requested approval from President Woolsey for a fund raising pamphlet and for a newly proposed plan of operation for the school. At the conclusion of this appeal to Woolsey, Ben said: 'With the good will and approbation of the Corporation, we shall have great hopes of success in our efforts . . . toward securing the expected endowment.'[139] Ben, Dana, and John A. Porter must have felt strongly the need for additional funding since they signed a note to the Yale Corporation for $500 in order to pay Daniel Coit Gilman's expenses as a fund raiser. They expected to repay this loan from the money Gilman raised. Some $25,000, an amount far below what was sought, was raised from the Yale and New Haven community, but the appeal probably helped to focus Joseph Sheffield's attention even more closely than before on the needs of the school; his $10,000 gift to the drive was soon increased many fold.

Benjamin Silliman, Jr. should be especially remembered for making two contributions to Yale's status as an international center for the study of science. The first was the founding in partnership with John Pitkin Norton of the Yale School of Applied Chemistry which soon flowered into the Sheffield Scientific School. The second was his role in securing the George Peabody endowment for the establishment

of the Peabody Museum. The original impetus for Peabody's gift of
$150,000 probably came from Benjamin Silliman, Sr. Silliman visited
Mr. Peabody in 1857 when Peabody came to Yale to see his nephew,
Othniel C. Marsh, then a student. Following this meeting, the elder
Silliman wrote Peabody to ask his support for the Scientific School.
Although no money was promised at that time, Benjamin Silliman was
one of the first to be informed when the great bequest was made, and he
was named by Peabody to be one of the original trustees of the Peabody
Museum.[140]

In 1862, Marsh, who had just completed two years of study in the
Sheffield Scientific School, wrote to Silliman, Jr., who had been one of
his teachers, to alert him to the fact that Marsh's uncle was prepared to
donate as much as $100,000 to Yale College. He asked Ben to suggest
how this money might be used.[141] There surely had been preliminary
discussions before the letter was sent, and probably 'Marsh's mentors,
James Dwight Dana and the younger Silliman, had . . . schooled him
in the logistics of scientific enterprise. . . .'[142] Ben discussed the news
with Dana, and both agreed that the best use of the bequest would be a
building with facilities for natural history, chemistry, physics, lecture
and recitation rooms, and a museum. They had once before proposed a
similar idea to another potential donor, without success.

Ben estimated that a building of the scope they envisaged would
require at least $150,000, and he suggested that it be called Peabody
Museum or Peabody Hall. 'It is so distinct,' he said, 'from the other
departments and outward presentments of the university that the name
of the Donor is sure to be always prominent and gratefully
remembered.'[143] A few months later the great news came. Marsh
announced to Benjamin Silliman, Sr. that Peabody definitely would
give $100,000, soon increased to $150,000, 'to promote the interests of
Natural Science' in Yale College. The trustees chosen by Peabody to
supervise the building and maintenance of the new museum were
Benjamin Silliman, Sr., James Dixon, James Dwight Dana, Benjamin
Silliman, Jr., and O. C. Marsh.[144]

Now something had to be done for Marsh, who was desperately
anxious to join the Yale faculty as professor of paleontology. Both
Benjamin Silliman, Jr. and James Dwight Dana were anxious to help,
and advised Marsh on his preparation for this position. Silliman, Jr.
was certain that as soon as Marsh showed his fitness, he would receive
the appointment. The most desirable thing, Ben urged, was to
persuade Mr. Peabody to endow the needed professorship.[145] Marsh,
although an expert at handling his uncle, did not secure the

endowment for his professorship. He told his uncle that he would need 'to have a library and cabinet in a measure equal to that possessed by my colleagues. A library and cabinet is to a Prof. of Science exactly what capital is to a man of business.' He urged him to give him $3-4,000 to spend in Europe for books and specimens. Both Silliman and Dana, he said, 'each have private libraries and cabinets of much greater value.'[146]

On 24 July 1866, after three years of advanced study in Europe, Marsh was appointed to the Chair of Palaeontology in the Scientific School, without salary.

Whether he was acting as a college teacher, a mining consultant, illuminating gas engineer, forensic chemist, or mineralogist, Ben kept in close touch with laboratory science. He was generally an excellent analyst, but he sometimes fell into error because he tended to depend on the work of students who were not supervised closely enough. George Brush, later an outstanding mineralogist and professor of mineralogy in the Sheffield Scientific School, testified to the lack of supervision in 1852:

> What an unfortunate paper that was that Silliman wrote the 1st year we were in the Labt on Emeryllite and etc. He, you know, formed 4 new species . . . only one of which will probably stand, the Clingmanite [Corundellite and Euphyllite] were proven to be identical with Emeryllite when we were in the Labt. All of these species or certainly the last three were made on Crooke's analyses but no man should *ever* make a new species on one analysis particularly on a student's analyses when he has not himself verified the results.[147]

Ben was not alone in creating new mineral species. Emeryllite, identified by J. Lawrence Smith, one of America's greatest nineteenth century mineralogist and chemists, turned out to be a variety of margarite and not a new species. The thousands of names one finds in the various mineralogies testify to the vast number of incorrectly identified mineral species. Silliman, Jr.'s 1849 paper was a disaster. Crook's analysis of Corundellite was erroneous since the amount of silica was incorrectly ascertained.[148] Yet Ben had cautiously remarked that 'this species somewhat resembles margarite. . . . Possibly a new analysis may bring these species together.'[149] The Clingmanite analysis also overestimated silica.[150] Ben recognized that he himself may have made an imperfect analysis because of an 'insufficient quantity of the mineral. . . . Should it appear on repeating the analysis of this mineral, that it is new, as the present would appear to indicate, I would propose to adopt the name *Clingmanite*, suggested by Prof. Shepard, in honor of the distinguished gentleman before named, who has shown great interest in advancing the study of mineralogy.'[151] Ben was also mistaken with Unionite, a variety of Zoisite, which he claimed was a new species.[152] His own analysis was seriously deficient in that it not only was too high in silica and aluminum, but he missed the mineral's iron and calcium completely, an astonishing error for a chemist of his experience.[153] Silliman, Jr.'s Monrolite was also troublesome to him for he hesitated to pronounce it as a new species because of its resemblance to Worthite. His analysis was defective with respect to silica and alumina. Monrolite was later identified as a variety of Sillimanite.[154]

These errors would seem to argue strongly that he was an incompetent mineralogical chemist. It is obvious that Ben could hardly wait to rush into print to secure priority, yet in other analyses reported in this paper, he was spectacularly correct. For example, he recognized that Sillimanite, Fibrolite, and Bucholzite were identical with Kyanite.[155] In this case, Ben's assistant was George J. Brush who, he said, 'afforded me essential aid.'[156] Brush also analyzed a specimen referred to as Indianite which Ben correctly decided was Anorthite.[157] Ben's decision to reestablish Boltonite as a mineral species was hasty. His analysis was high on silica and low on magnesia. Boltonite turned out to be a variety of Forsterite.[158] Ludwig Stadtmuller, who later worked for Ben as a mining engineer, analyzed nuttallite. Stadtmuller's analysis was excellent, and Ben's conclusion that nuttallite was a scopolite was correct.[159] Despite his errors, most of Ben's extensive analytical work on minerals was of a high enough quality to be cited in Dana's *System of Mineralogy* throughout the nineteenth century.[160]

A few years earlier, Ben had been embarrassed because, in a scientific paper read in 1844 to the Association of American Geologists and Naturalists, James Dwight Dana relied on an erroneous analysis of Ben's. Dana, citing the large percentage of phosphoric acid, up to 9 or 10%, which Ben had found in corals, proceeded from this fact to an analogy between the chemical structure of higher animals and of coral.[161] Dana went on to infer that primary limestones and dolomites were 'altered sedimentary limestones and that these limestones may be, in part, of coral origin.'[162] Ben apologized for this earlier work in a footnote to one of his most important papers:

> In vol. XLVII, p. 135, of this Journal, some earlier results obtained by me on this subject were stated, which were prematurely published, and

greatly erroneous. . . . The best antidote to an error of this sort is the early publication of correct and trustworthy results. It is to be hoped that the researches detailed in this paper are of this description, and the attention of those interested in such studies is invited to the repetition of the analyses here given. The geological interest of these observations is not in any way lessened by the results recently obtained, although differing so much from those previously published.[163]

In this study, Ben reported the results of nearly three years of work on the analysis of the coral specimens brought back by Dana from the Wilkes Expedition. It summarizes research which was also published in Dana's monumental treatise on zoophytes, of which only 200 copies were issued. In this paper, as was his custom, he warmly thanked his assistants, Denison Olmsted, Jr. and T. S. Hunt, for their help.[164] The work seems to have been extraordinarily good. It has been cited recently by Levorsen, who emphasized its significance in understanding the origin of petroleum. Silliman was the first to show that corals contain organic matter, and a fatty waxlike residue, soluble in ether, but insoluble in alcohol.[165] Ben wrote in 1846 that this wax '. . . deserves more attention than I have been able to give it.'[166]

In 1922 Clarke and Wheeler carefully reviewed many reported coral analyses and compared them with their own analyses made with better techniques. They accepted Silliman's analyses without question, adding that 'the uniformity of the data is so marked that it is unnecessary to reproduce all the published analyses here.'[167] Some ninety years after its publication, Bergmann and Lester, two Yale scientists, paid special attention to Silliman, Jr.'s classical paper in their treatment of modes of petroleum formation. They called it a pioneering work and noted that 'since Silliman's time practically no work has been done on the organic constituents in corals, which is rather surprising because the reef-building corals occur in almost unlimited abundance in the coastal regions of tropical waters.'[168] They repeated and confirmed Silliman's analyses, although with much greater accuracy and better identification of constituents. They also confirmed Ben's conclusion that 'this organic matter is . . . intimately united throughout the whole structure of the corals.'[169]

In addition to the corals the younger Silliman analyzed a variety of mineral and rock specimens from the Wilkes Expedition. He was less successful with these, and few of his analyses have stood the test of time. His analysis of Pele's hair, a glassy scoria from the Kilauea Volcano, and two minerals which he hastily named as new species, *Mauilite* and *Samoite* were in error.[170] The Samoite which he analyzed late in 1848 in the Analytical Laboratory seems to have been based on only one analysis.[171] It was dismissed by Dana as 'a kind of feldspar incorrectly analyzed, probably laboradorite.'[172]

Although Benjamin Silliman, Jr.'s work on the Kilauea specimens was of dubious quality, Dana continued to rely on his coral analyses, and the analyses of coral sands and chalk from an Oahu reef.[173] Dana never criticized Ben directly in his published work. Edward Salisbury Dana, his son, was somewhat more forthright. Many years later, following a series of analyses of the Kilauea lavas, he wrote: 'The remark made by Professor J. D. Dana must be repeated here that the early analyses published in the Geological Report of the U.S. Exploring Expedition, having been made for him by an inexperienced analyst, are entirely unreliable and should not be quoted.'[174] James Dwight Dana's criticism was much less direct even though it appeared after Silliman died, and some fifty years after the faulty analyses:[175] 'I add that I do not cite here the analyses of the rocks and volcanic glass of Kilauea made by another for me and published in my Expedition report, because they are erroneous and should be rejected.'[176]

Ben attained a high reputation as a water chemist. His work with the Boston waters in 1845 was excellent. The water commissioners compared his results with those of such well-known chemists as Augustus A. Gould, S. L. Dana, Charles T. Jackson, and Eben N. Horsford and were well satisfied: 'We engaged the services of Benjamin Silliman, Jr. Esq. whose skill and ability is, and the stores of whose well provided laboratory, have enabled him with promptitude to complete the desired researches and to make the report which we have the pleasure to present.'[177]

The analysis, with the assistance of Hunt and Olmsted, of a series of bottled water samples whose origin Ben did not know occupied some thirty working days. In 1849, Dr. M. Boyé, in a paper entitled 'On the Composition of the Schuylkill Water' compared his own analyses with those which Ben had obtained from Schuylkill water samples. Their results agreed closely.[178] Since the men and women of Yale regard only one other institution as possibly worthy of comparison with Yale, it is noteworthy that when the mineral cabinet at Harvard was in a shambles, Benjamin Silliman, Jr. was commissioned to put it into order, a task which took some two weeks.[179]

Despite Bache's doubts about his competence, Ben was elected to the important Standing Committee of the American Association for the Advancement of Science six times during its first fourteen years of existence. Bache himself served eleven times on this committee, Dana, seven, Benjamin Peirce, six, and Joseph Henry, five.[180]

Silliman's rock oil report of 1855 has long been famous. He possessed real competence as an oil chemist. A group of New Haven businessmen, considering the possibility of financing a company formed to sell petroleum, asked him to analyze oil samples, and to predict whether or not the oil was commercially useful. They considered him 'that mentor of all that was scientific in New Haven.'[181]

The oil report has been both criticized and praised. R. J. Forbes, a noted petroleum historian, has commented that Ben failed to apply 'the new theories of the organic chemists' to his research and that he was unaware of the research on petroleum which had been underway for years in Europe.[182] The charge is hardly credible because Ben received all the major European publications by exchange with the *Journal*. He has also been accused of knowing little about European production of lubricants from crude oil.[183] His report did not cover a number of products and uses for mineral oils which had already been proposed by others, and he was criticized for oversimplifying the preparation of a satisfactory illuminant from crude oil.[184] Williamson remarks: 'Even as late as 1860, his endorsement of defecated whale oil as "unsurpassed" as a lubricant does not suggest a very profound knowledge of this phase of the subject.' Williamson's comment referred to the following advertisement in the *Scientific American*:

> DEFECATED OIL - Railroad managers, engineers, machinists, etc. will find in this oil the long sought lubricator. It is manufactured from whale oil, and contains no mixture of any other oil or any other substance. It neither attacks nor corrodes the metal. It withstands more heat, more cold than any other oil, and is always uniform in quality. In a long report by Professor Silliman of Yale College, he writes—1st, That as a lubricator, the defecated oil stand unrivaled. That in its capacity to withstand changes of temperature, and causes which result in 'gumming up' it is unrivaled. Sold by BILLINGS AND MARSH, New London, Conn.[185]

Silliman, Jr. was surely not very wrong. Whale oil is still unsurpassed for certain types of lubrication.

Despite his criticisms, Williamson says that 'perhaps the most epochal report on petroleum history was made available when Eveleth personally succeeded in raising the money to meet Silliman's bid.'[186] The report had its shortcomings, but it 'was a landmark in its timeless and critical perceptions of petroleum's possibilities.'[187] Ben's most valuable insight was that new products could be formed by 'cracking' crude oil. Soon after 1855 Silliman Jr.'s deduction was put into practice by refiners who were cracking petroleum long before Berthelot published his findings, probably as early as 1858 by Downer's Kerosene Oil Co.[188]

Ben is mentioned twice in Darmstaedter's *Compendium of Scientific Discoveries.* For the year 1855 he is cited for 'the first petroleum lamp with a wick and a tension cylinder.'[189] For 1860 he is cited for establishing 'the anomalous boiling point of hydrocarbons of petroleum and [concluding] that a part of these hydrocarbons are not original constituents of petroleum but are formed by "cleavage" during distillation.' This view was confirmed in 1861 in a Newark refinery by the observation that 'hydrocarbons of petroleum are decomposed by contact with the hot walls of the distillation apparatus.'[190] The 1860 date is curious since the ideas referred to were enunciated in Ben's 1855 paper.[191]

The rock oil report has been reprinted at least six times and was included in such important works as Ida Tarbell's *History of the Standard Oil Co.* In 1955 it was reissued as a pamphlet by the Ethyl Corporation. Books on petroleum published in the late nineteenth century give him and his report respectful treatment: 'this distinguished chemist [who] made an exceedingly interesting and valuable report to the company' and 'this highly satisfactory report from such a distinguished source.'[192]

Some years later, when oil well production was already enormous, and after a visit to the oil regions and to some refineries in Cleveland, Silliman wrote: 'Some of our ingenious fellows will yet make a fortune from the discovery of a mode of utilizing the waste products [from preparing "naptha and light oils"] . . . Especially of the *light oils* forming fully one third of the gross product and for which there is hardly any use, being too volatile to use safely in lamps.'[193] He referred here to the gasoline fraction which, with the development of the gasoline motor, would eventually be in great demand.

Although Ben was guilty of careless work on several occasions, it is clear that he was capable of excellent work when he had time, or when something particularly interested him. His work on meteorites, on the daguerreotype, and on improvements in gas illumination all were of great interest. Ben was later criticized by Josiah D. Whitney and W. H. Brewer for his optimistic statements about California oil and for the gold mining interests from which he made (and lost) a great deal of money. His activities in these fields and the fact that he lent his name to speculations of various kinds caused the severe difficulties he experienced from the middle of the 1860s to almost the end of his life. This aspect of his life is well described in White's *Scientists in Conflict* as is his partial vindication. 'Professor Silliman had been responsible in considerable measure for his own troubles. In his reports on oil, for example, he had been rash, uncritical, overenthusiastic, and far too trusting of men who were not scientists.'[194]

Throughout Benjamin Silliman, Jr.'s life his enthusiasm and trust caused him endless trouble, because he was eternally involved in business deals of various kinds. His scientific critics were men who, in a later period, concentrated on pure science and 'were particularly distressed by the widespread corruption and crude materialism of the post-Civil War era. While not necessarily accepting all of Whitney's charges, they were willing to believe that Silliman had been false to his trust as a scientist and had damaged the good name of science before the world.'[195]

But Benjamin Silliman, Jr. was not the only professor who profited from commercial pursuits. Spence notes that 'Professors in colleges across the land found "experting" a welcome (and profitable) break from the routine of campus life. . . . Probably the majority of mining, mineralogy, and metallurgy professors did some examining of western property.'[196] Ben was surely not the most trusting and optimistic of these experts who as a group, because they were often wrong, were frequently involved in lawsuits. Since speculators were not especially scrupulous, they often selected only the most favorable sections of reports, rejected unfavorable reports, and continued to use reports after the mining properties concerned had been proven to be worthless. Ben complained in 1877 that a mining prospectus based on an 1864 report he had written was still in use as late as 1877 'although subsequent exploration had been negative.'[197]

Silliman, Jr. was proud of his role as a scientific expert and was often called to testify in lawsuits when expert scientific testimony was required:

> It is possible for the man of real science, and skilled in his art, to confer great benefit, not only upon the parties of interest, but upon the subject; while science itself often gains by the researches which are called out by these contests upon which have before been overlooked or imperfectly investigated. I have been frequently called upon to testify as an expert in cases requiring scientific testimony.[198]

One of Silliman's collaborators in gaslighting research, H. E. Sadler, wrote a splendid memorial which was published soon after Ben died:

> [He] was in no sense a leader of scientific thought. He had hit upon no
> such discoveries as those by which Henry opened the way for the telegraph
> or by which Bell had produced the telephone. He had not pushed
> speculation to the limit of human reason. He had not been the founder of
> any school of philosophy. Even in his chosen field of chemistry, it has
> fallen to his colleagues, to Cooke, to Gibbs, to Lawrence Smith, to extend
> the written laws of nature and make the broader generalization.
>
> What he has accomplished . . . will be appreciated only by those who
> know how manifold were his interests outside of science, by those who
> have learned the prodigality with which he bestowed his time upon his
> pupils, by those who remember his remarkable faithfulness to the hum-
> blest duties, even self-imposed.[199]

In the end, despite the sorrows of his later life, Silliman, Jr.'s
inborn optimism, his ingenuousness and simplicity, his capacity for
making friends, for forgiving those who attacked him, and for suffer-
ing without resort to the same mean and bitter attacks, and his
magnanimity of spirit allowed him to rise above his accusers. One
prefers to think of him as a genial professor and not as the conniving
entrepreneur:

> To have access to Prof. Silliman's study was to lay the foundations of
> character. It was to make all lovely things seem still more lovely, to learn
> the worth of easy circumstance, of domestic peace, of gentle sympathy, of
> devotion to duty, of learning, manners, and modesty, of simplicity when
> fortune smiles, of unswerving fortitude when she frowns. His library was a
> large room, blending by ample baywindow with the garden. Its stretch of
> floor was broken by thick and kindly rugs, by escritoire and reading desk,
> by map cases, easels, and quaint chairs. Its mantel over-arched a grate of
> flaming coal which cast a glow like the peaceful love that reigned there.
> Piled high around were line after line and tier after tier of scientific
> periodicals and books, most cherished if not sole return from a half a
> century's devotion to the *American Journal*. The sustained and serious,
> but bright and cheerful, occupation of the family, the earnest but above all
> kindly face of the master, complete a picture such as we love to hang on
> memory's wall.[200]

NOTES

[1] Josiah P. Cooke, 'Benjamin Silliman,' *Proc. Am. Acad. Arts Sci.*, 1885, *20*, 526.

[2] Dwight, *Memories of Yale Life and Men*, p. 364.

[3] Silliman, Jr. to wife, 25 December 1864, Silliman Family Papers.

[35] Silliman to Silliman, Jr., 3 December 1849, Silliman Family Papers.

[36] Silliman, Jr. to wife, 5 January 1851, Silliman Family Papers.

[37] Silliman, Jr. to Brewer, 31 January 1853, Brewer Papers.

[38] Brush to Brewer, 19 April 1851, Brewer Papers.

[39] *Ibid.*, 30 November 1851.

[40] *Ibid.*, 24 October 1850.

[41] Silliman to Silliman, Jr., 16 November 1849, Silliman Family Papers.

[42] Walter B. Hendrickson, 'Museums and Natural History Societies in Louisville,' *Filson Club hist. Quart.*, 1962, *36*, 44.

[43] Eliot Jarvis to Brewer, 30 November 1851, Brewer Papers.

[44] Silliman, Jr. to wife, 5 January 1851, Silliman Family Papers.

[45] Silliman to Silliman, Jr., 18 November 1850, Silliman Family Papers.

[46] H. E. Sadler, 'Prof. Benjamin Silliman, Jr., '*Kans. Cy Rev. Sci. Ind.*, March 1885, p. 4.

[47] Maria Trumbull Dana, 'Hillhouse Avenue,' paper read in 1930 to the Saturday Morning Club, Dana Family Papers.

[48] Silliman, Jr. to wife, 8 January 1851, Silliman Family Papers.

[49] Silliman, *Am. J. Sci.*, 1847, *50*, Preface, pp. xiii–xiv.

[50] Joseph Henry to Alexander D. Bache, in Reingold, ed., *Science in Nineteenth Century America*, pp. 84–85.

[51] Silliman, 'Personal Notices,' X, unpaged, 20 July 1845, Silliman Family Papers.

[52] Alexander D. Bache to John Fries Frazer, 12 March 1863, Frazer Papers.

[53] 'Minutes of the Prudential Committee,' 26 December 1843.

[54] Silliman to Silliman, Jr., undated but probably toward end of 1849, Silliman Family Papers.

[55] Silliman, Jr. to Gideon A. Mantell, 29 April 1846, Silliman Family Papers.

[56] Silliman to Silliman, Jr. undated but probably toward end of 1849, Silliman Family Papers.

[57] 'Agreement' between Benjamin Silliman, Sr., Benjamin Silliman, Jr., and James Dwight Dana, 5 December 1850, Dana Family Papers.

[58] Silliman, 'Probate Court Record,' 6 June 1873, Connecticut State Library, Probate Record Section, Hartford, Connecticut.

[59] 'Agreement,' Silliman, Jr. with James Dwight Dana, 18 May 1878, Silliman Family Papers.

[60] Silliman to Silliman, Jr. undated but probably end of 1849, Silliman Family Papers.

[61] Silliman, Jr. to Lunsford P. Yandell, 5 June 1850, Silliman Family Papers.

[62] Silliman, Jr. to Brewer, 31 January 1854, Brewer Papers.

[63] Mason Weld to Silliman, Jr., 31 July 1854, Silliman Family Papers.

[64] Silliman, 'Letter Book, with copies of many of his letters, 1851–1869,' 11 February 1853, Silliman Family Papers.

Louis I. Kuslan

Silliman, 'Personal Notices,' pp. 80–83, Silliman Family Paper

Davis, *Chronicles of Hopkins Grammar School*, p. 313.

James Hall to Silliman, Jr., 15 January 1840; James Hall to Silli Silliman Family Papers.

Barnett F. Dodge, in Ethyl Corporation, *Benjamin Silliman, Jr*

Silliman, Jr. to Brewer, 1 February 1854, Brewer Papers.

Silliman, Jr. to wife, 10 January 1840, Silliman Family Papers.

'Day Book,' Treasurer's Accounts, Yale College, Yale Univer entries for 26 January, 24 April and 17 August 1838; 1 January, 22 Ap 19 December 1839.

'Minutes of the Prudential Committee,' 26 December 1843 and University Archives.

Silliman to wife, 8 January 1835, Silliman Family Papers.

Silliman, 'Personal Notices,' VI, (1 January - 15 May 1842) unpaged, Silliman Family Papers.

Margaret W. Rossiter, 'Benjamin Silliman and the Lowell Institu zation of Science in Nineteenth Century America,' *New Engl. Quart.,*

Silliman, 'Personal Notices,' XI, unpaged, 24 April 1845, Sillim;

Fisher, *Silliman*, I, 362–363.

Susan Forbes Silliman to Gideon Mantell, 25 June 1845, Sillim;

Silliman, 'Laboratory Blotter,' 1843–44, p. 372, Silliman Family

Louis I. Kuslan, 'The Founding of the Yale School of Applied C *Med.*, 1969, *24*, 430–451.

Silliman, Jr. to Oliver P. Hubbard, 2 February 1838, Silliman F

Silliman to Silliman, Jr., 21 October 1840, Silliman Family Pap

Silliman, 'Laboratory Blotter,' 11 November 1840, Silliman Fan

Ibid., 21 October 1841.

Ibid., 5 January 1842.

Ibid., 17 November 1847.

Silliman, 'Personal Notices,' XIII, unpaged, 28 September 1849, Papers.

Ibid., XI, unpaged, 9 November 1845.

Ibid., X, unpaged, 30 May 1845.

James Dwight Dana to Augustus A. Gould, 9 February 1846, Dan This letter was brought to my attention by Michael Prendergast.

Silliman, Jr. to wife, 26 January 1847, Silliman Family Papers.

Silliman, 'Personal Notices,' XIII, unpaged, 15 April 1849, Papers.

Ibid., 22 April and 7 May 1849.

Silliman to Gideon Mantell, 1 March 1849, Silliman Family Pap

Silliman, 'Personal Notices,' X, unpaged, 15 April 1849, Sillimar

[65] O. C. Marsh to G. P. Peabody, 7 July 1863 in Schuchert and Levene, *Marsh*, p. 53.

[66] *Ibid.*, p. 54.

[67] Silliman to Silliman, Jr., 26 February 1853, Silliman Family Papers.

[68] Silliman, Jr. to Brewer, 1 February 1854, Silliman Family Papers.

[69] Silliman to Silliman, Jr., 26 February 1853, Silliman Family Papers.

[70] *Ibid.*, 16 January 1854.

[71] 'Minutes of the Yale Corporation,' 26 July 1853, p. 71, Yale University Archives.

[72] Silliman, Jr., 'Address to the 1854 Louisville Medical Department Graduates,' Silliman Family Papers.

[73] 'Minutes of the Yale Corporation,' July 1856, p. 312.

[74] Silliman to Silliman, Jr., 16 January 1854, Silliman Family Papers.

[75] Silliman, Jr. to President and Fellows, 8 May 1854, Silliman Family Papers.

[76] 'Minutes of the Prudential Committee,' 27 July 1855.

[77] Margaret Rossiter, 'Justus Liebig and the Americans,' p. 18.

[78] C. A. Browne, 'The History of Chemical Education in America Between the Years 1820 and 1870,' *J. Chem. Educ.*, 1932, *9*, 724.

[79] Silliman to Gideon A. Mantell, 24 February 1847, Silliman Family Papers.

[80] Fownes, *Elementary Chemistry*.

[81] Silliman, Jr., *First Principles of Chemistry*, Preface.

[82] Silliman, Jr. to Brewer, 31 January 1853, Brewer Papers.

[83] *Ibid.*, 10 January 1859.

[84] *Ibid.*, 25 February 1859.

[85] *Ibid.*, 7 March 1859.

[86] *Dictionary of Scientific Biography*, s.v., 'Silliman, Jr., Benjamin.'

[87] Joseph Willet to Brewer, 25 November 1852, Brewer Papers.

[88] *Ibid.*

[89] Kelley, *Yale*, p. 179.

[90] Silliman to Silliman, Jr., 6 December 1849, Silliman Family Papers.

[91] George P. Brush to Brewer, 2 February 1851, Brewer Papers.

[92] *Ibid.*, 30 November 1851.

[93] *Ibid.*, 2 February 1851.

[94] See White, *Scientists in Conflict* for details.

[95] Silliman, Jr. to Brewer, 13 July 1858, Brewer Papers.

[96] *Ibid.*, 24 January 1863.

[97] Merrill, *The First One Hundred Years of American Geology*, pp. 447–448.

[98] Silliman, 'Personal Notes,' XIII, unpaged, 10 September 1848, Silliman Family Papers.

[99] T. Sterry Hunt, 'Biographical Notice of Benjamin Silliman.' *Trans. Am. Inst. Min. Engrs.*, 1885, *13*, 783.

[100] Silliman, Jr., *First Principles of Chemistry*, Preface.

[101] For Enri's life see W. D. Miles and L. I. Kuslan, 'Washington's First Consulting Chemist, Henri Erni,' in Rosenberger, ed., *Columbia Historical Society*, pp. 154–166.

[102] *Proc. Am. Ass. Advmt. Sci.*, 1850, p. 383.

[103] 'New Haven City Gas Light Charter.'

[104] Henry H. Townshend, 'The Formative Years of New Haven's Public Utilities,' in Kirby, ed., *Inventors and Engineers*, p. 55.

[105] *Ibid.*, p. 58.

[106] Record Book of New Haven Gas Light Company, p. 7.

[107] Silliman, Jr. and Goodrich, eds., *World of Science, Art and Industry*, p. vii.

[108] *Ibid.*, pp. 59–76.

[109] *Ibid.*, p. 20.

[110] Silliman, Jr., 'Report on the Breckenridge Coal, 9 February 1854,' in *Charter of the Breckenridge Cannel Coal Co., Granted by the General Assembly of Kentucky* (place and date of publication not given). Copy in the Yale Archives.

[111] Silliman and Silliman, Jr., *Extracts From a Report Made to the Maryland and New York Coal Company*.

[112] Silliman, Jr. to wife, 20 February 1864. Except during academic terms, Ben was away more than he was at home. This habit had begun before his marriage, and was so strong that Susan once remarked poignantly 'You are so much away from home.' Susan Forbes Silliman to Silliman, Jr., 12 March 1841 or 1842, Silliman Family Papers.

[113] Silliman, Jr., *Descriptive Notice of the Steam Heating Apparatus*, p. 18. Jonathan Knight, professor of surgery in the Yale Medical Department and a member of the board of this company, also wrote an enthusiastic recommendation.

[114] *Ibid.*, p. 17.

[115] *Remarks of Prof. B. Silliman, Jr. Before a Committee of the Board of Education of New York*.

[116] Silliman, Jr. to wife, 2 December 1866, Silliman Family Papers.

[117] 'Sketch of Benjamin Silliman,' *Pop. Sci. Mon.*, 1880, *16*, 551, reprinted from Kingsley, *Yale College*.

[118] Rossiter, *Emergence of Agricultural Science*, pp. 19, 96.

[119] See Sally G. Kohlstedt's paper, 'The Geologist's Model for National Science,' *Proc. Am. phil. Soc.*, 1974, *118*, 179–195, for additional details about young Silliman's role in this association.

[120] Silliman, Jr., *Report on the Rock Oil*.

[121] Lawrence, *Pet oleum Comes of Age*, p. 67.

[122] White, *Scientists in Conflict*, p. 43.

[123] *Ibid.*; M. L. Norton, 'Copper Mines in Bristol,' in *Bristol, Connecticut*, p. 441.

[124] Silliman, Jr. and Whitney, *Bristol Copper Mine*, p. 12.

[125] Peck, *History of Bristol, Connecticut*, p. 137.

[126] White, *Scientists in Conflict*, p. 43.

[127] Norton (n. 123).

[128] Peck, *History of Bristol, Connecticut*, p. 137.

[129] E. M. Hulbert, 'Copper Mining in Connecticut,' *Conn. Mag.*, 1897, *3*, 27.

[130] *Ibid.* p. 27.

[131] Cited in Charles K. Harte, 'Connecticut's Iron and Copper,' *Rep. Conn. Soc. civ. Engrs.*, 1944, *60*, 152. This report appeared in *The Bristol Herald*, 15 August 1889.

[132] Silliman, Jr., 'Testimony,' pp. 39-40.

[133] *Ibid.*, p. 4.

[134] Printed flyer citing Benjamin Silliman, Jr.'s Report on the F. R. Slocum Marble Quarry in Falls Village, Ct., 1855.

[135] 'Minutes of the Prudential Committee,' 30 July 1844.

[136] Kohlstedt (n. 119), p. 187.

[137] 'Minutes of the Prudential Committee,' 19 July 1854.

[138] Cited in Kuslan (n. 19), p. 440.

[139] Dana and Silliman, Jr. to Pres. Theodore Woolsey, 11 July 1858, Woolsey Family Papers.

[140] Schuchert and Levene, *Marsh*, p. 13.

[141] *Ibid.*, p. 75.

[142] Miller, *Dollars for Research*, p. 139.

[143] Schuchert and Levene, *Marsh*, p. 75.

[144] *Ibid.*, p. 85. The authors are in error on the matter of Ben's service on the Peabody Museum Board of Trustees. They state that Ben did not serve on the board '. . . since he left Yale to teach Chemistry at Louisville, Kentucky.' Silliman, Jr. ended his service in Louisville in 1854, and he continued as a Peabody trustee until his death.

[145] *Ibid.*, p. 51.

[146] *Ibid.*, p. 54.

[147] George P. Brush to Brewer, 28 November 1852, Brewer Papers.

[148] Dana, *System of Mineralogy*, 6th ed., pp. 636-637.

[149] Silliman, Jr., 'Descriptions and Analyses of Several American Minerals,' *Am. J. Sci.*, 1849, *2nd ser. 8*, 381.

[150] Dana, *System of Mineralogy*, 6th ed., p. 632.

[151] Silliman, Jr., (n. 149), p. 383.

[152] Dana, *System of Mineralogy*, 6th ed., p. 513.

[153] Silliman, Jr., (n. 149), p. 385.

[154] Dana, *System of Mineralogy*, 6th ed., p. 499.

[155] Silliman, Jr., (n. 149), p. 389. Dana's *System of Mineralogy*, 6th ed., notes on pp. 498-500 that Sillimanite, Fibrolite, and Bucholzite are varieties of Sillimanite, and that Cyanite is a closely related species.

[156] Silliman, Jr. (n. 149), p. 389.

[157] *Ibid.*, p. 391.

[158] *Ibid.*, p. 393.

[159] Dana, *System of Mineralogy*, 6th ed., p. 469.

[160] See, for example, in Dana, *System of Mineralogy*, 5th ed., pp. 8, 41, 177, 178, 299, 303, 304, 306, 312, 313, 359, 374, 419, 420, 506, 507, 747, 748.

[161] James Dwight Dana, 'On the Composition of Corals and the Production of the Phosphates, Aluminates, Silicates, and other minerals, by the Metamorphic Action of Hot Water,' *Am. J. Sci.*, 1844, *47*, 135-136.

[162] *Ibid.*, p. 135.

[163] Silliman, Jr., 'On the Chemical Composition of the Calcareous Corals,' *Am. J. Sci.*, 1846, *2nd ser. 1*, 189.

[164] *Ibid.*, p. 199.

[165] Levorsen, *Geology of Petroleum*, p. 488.

[166] Silliman, Jr. (n. 163), p. 197.

[167] Clarke et al., *Inorganic Constituents of Marine Invertebrates*, p. 9. Silliman's was the oldest paper cited in this study, the others ranging from 1852 to 1922.

[168] Warner Bergmann and David Lester, 'Coral-Reefs and the Formation of Petroleum,' *Science*, 1940, *92*, 452-453.

[169] Silliman, Jr. (n. 163), p. 197.

[170] Dana, *Geology*, pp. 230, 732.

[171] Yale Analytical Laboratory 'Record Book,' pp. 13-14, Sheffield Records.

[172] Dana, *System of Mineralogy*, 5th ed., p. 478.

[173] Dana, *Corals and Coral Islands*, pp. 394-395.

[174] Edward S. Dana, 'Contributions to the Petrography of the Sandwich Islands,' *Am. J. Sci.*, 1889, *36*, 462.

[175] Edward S. Dana seems to have shared the dislike for Ben exhibited by many of his colleagues in the Sheffield Scientific School. The few references to Silliman's work in Dana's *Century of Science* is a case in point. His comment is repeated in James Dwight Dana's *Characteristics of Volcanoes*, p. 347 in the chapter on the petrography of the Hawaiian Islands which he wrote. James Dwight Dana may have agreed for he allowed it to appear unchanged.

[176] James D. Dana, 'A History of the Changes in Kilauea,' *Am. J. Sci.*, 1888, *35*, 223.

[177] Boston. [Water] Commissioners, *Report*, p. 95.

[178] Martin H. Boyé, 'On the Composition of the Schuylkill Waters,' *Proc. Am. Ass. Advmt Sci.*, 1849, pp. 123-132.

[179] Silliman, 'Personal Notices,' XIV, 330, 18 July 1852, Silliman Family Papers.

[180] Daniels, *Science in American Society*, p. 169.

[181] Townshend, *New Haven and the First Oil Well*, p. 3.

[182] Forbes, *Early Petroleum History*, pp. 63-64.

[183] Robert J. Forbes, 'Petroleum,' in Singer et al., eds., *History of Technology*, V. 109.

[184] Williamson and Daum, *American Petroleum Industry*, p. 71.

[185] *Scient. Am.*, 1860, *2*, 399.

[186]Williamson and Daum, *American Petroleum Industry*, p. 69.

[187]*Ibid.*, p. 71.

[188]*Ibid.*, pp. 205, 219.

[189]Ludwig Darmstaedter, *Geschichte der Naturwissenschaften*, pp. 560–561.

[190]*Ibid.*, p. 188.

[191]It is interesting that the American Association for the Advancement of Science publication by Lark-Horovitz and Carmichael, *Chronology of Scientific Development*, makes the same error.

[192]Crow, *Practical Treatise on Petroleum*, pp. 136–139.

[193]Silliman, Jr. to wife, 2 December 1866, Silliman Family Papers.

[194]See White, *Scientists in Conflict*, ch. 8 in particular.

[195]*Ibid.*, pp. 229–230.

[196]Spence, *Mining Engineers*, p. 85.

[197]*Ibid.*, p. 118.

[198]Silliman, Jr., 'Testimony,' preface and p. 3.

[199]Sadler, (n. 46), p. 1.

[200]*Ibid.*, p. 3.

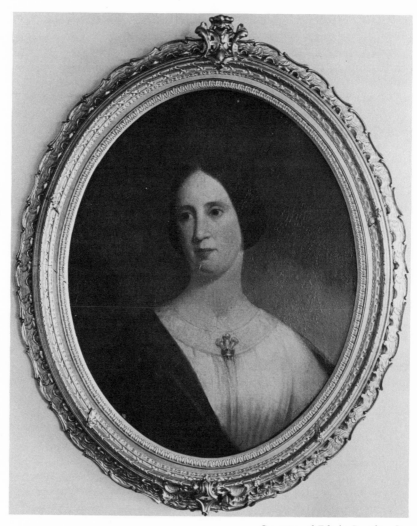

Courtesy of Edwin Pugsley, Jr.

Susan Forbes Silliman

Manuscript Sources

Blake Family Papers. Yale University Library. New Haven, Connecticut.

William Henry Brewer Papers. Yale University Library. New Haven, Connecticut.

Brush Family Papers. Yale University Library. New Haven, Connecticut. The Brush collection contains about thirty letters from James Dwight Dana to George Brush, 1852-56, mostly about mineralogy and the Yale Scientific School. It also contains over seventy letters from Henrietta Dana to Harriet Trumbull from 1851 on.

Parker Cleaveland Correspondence. Bowdoin College Library. Brunswick, Maine.

Dana Family Papers. Yale University Library. New Haven, Connecticut. The Dana collection contains extensive family and scientific correspondence.

J. W. De Forest Family Papers. Collection of American Literature. Beinecke Rare Book and Manuscript Library. Yale University. New Haven, Connecticut.

John Fries Fraser Papers. American Philosophical Society. Philadelphia, Pennsylvania.

Gibbs Family Papers. Newport Historical Society. Newport, Rhode Island. Contain extensive correspondence from scientific associates of Colonel Gibbs, including letters of Silliman, Maclure, Eaton, Cleaveland, Torrey, Gilmore, and Rafinesque. Miscellaneous materials include lists of minerals.

Gibbs Family Papers. State Historical Society of Wisconsin. Madison, Wisconsin. Contain papers of George Gibbs, IV (1815-73), some early correspondence of his father, Colonel Gibbs, and accounts and letters of Oliver Wolcott.

Mary Channing Gibbs (1747-1824) trust estate, financial records. New York Historical Society, New York, New York.

Edward C. Herrick Papers. Yale University Library. New Haven, Connecticut. Contain sixty-five letters to and from James Dwight Dana, 1832-45, concerning Dana's travels and scientific matters at Yale.

Francis Bernard Higgins Papers. Amherst College Library. Amherst, Massachusetts.

President Edward Hitchcock Papers. Amherst College Library. Amherst, Massachusetts.

S. W. Johnson Manuscripts. Connecticut Agricultural Experiment Station. New Haven, Connecticut.

Elias Loomis Papers. Beinecke Rare Book and Manuscript Library. Yale University. New Haven, Connecticut. Contain nine letters from James Dwight Dana, mostly about Loomis's contributions to the *American Journal of Science*.

Othniel Charles Marsh Papers. Yale University Library. New Haven, Connecticut. Contain about sixty letters from James Dwight Dana, all of which are on microfilm.

Mineralogical Papers, 1824–1934. Department of Geology. Yale University Archives. Yale University Library. New Haven, Connecticut. Consists of four boxes. The first contains much Silliman and Dana correspondence about the mineral collections at Yale.

'Minutes of the Prudential Committee.' Yale University Archives. Yale University Library. New Haven, Connecticut.

'Minutes of the Yale Corporation.' Yale University Archives. Yale University Library. New Haven, Connecticut.

New Haven City Gas Light Charter. Doc. no. 1918. Southern Connecticut Gas Company, Bridgeport, Connecticut.

John Pitkin Norton Papers. Yale University Library. New Haven, Connecticut.

Benjamin Peirce Papers. Houghton Library, Harvard University. Cambridge, Massachusetts.

James Gates Percival Papers. Collection of American Literature. Beinecke Rare Book and Manuscript Library, Yale University. New Haven, Connecticut.

Record Book of New Haven Gas Light Company. Southern Connecticut Gas Company. Bridgeport, Connecticut.

William C. Redfield Papers. Beinecke Rare Book and Manuscript Library, Yale University. New Haven, Connecticut. Contain nineteen letters from James Dwight Dana, 1838–57, on meteorology, ocean currents, and Wilkes Expedition as well as letters from other scientists.

Sheffield Scientific School Records. Yale University Archives, Yale University Library. New Haven, Connecticut.

Charles Upham Shepard materials. Waring Historical Library. Medical University of South Carolina. Charleston, South Carolina.

Charles Upham Shepard Papers. Amherst College Library. Amherst, Massachusetts.

Silliman Family Papers. Yale University Library. New Haven, Connecticut.
    Include: 'Origin and Progress in chemistry, mineralogy, and geology in Yale College and in other places, with personal reminiscences,' 9 vols. [1857–62]; referred to as 'Reminiscences.' 'Personal Notices or private journals, 1840–1864,' 17 vols.

Treasurer's Accounts, Yale College. Yale University Archives, Yale University Library. New Haven, Connecticut. Include 'Day Book.'

Wolcott-Gibbs Family Papers. University of Oregon. Eugene, Oregon. Contain some seventy Gibbs family letters, primarily between family members.

Woolsey Family Papers. Yale University Archives, Yale University. New Haven, Connecticut.

Bibliography

American Antiquarian Society. *Proceedings, 1812-1849*. Worcester, Mass.: The Society, 1912.

Amherst College. *Biographical Record of the Alumni of Amherst College, During its First Half Century: 1821-1871*. Edited by W. L. Montague. Amherst, Mass.: 1883.

Beckham, Stephen D. 'George Gibbs IV: Historian and Ethnologist.' Ph.D. dissertation, University of California-Los Angeles, 1969.

Bixby, William. *The Forgotten Voyage of Charles Wilkes*. New York: D. McKay Co., 1966.

Boston. Commissioners to examine the sources from which pure water may be obtained. *Report*. Boston: J. H. Eastburn, 1845.

Bristol, Connecticut ('In the Olden Time New Cambridge') which includes Forestville. Hartford, Conn.: City Print. Company, 1907.

Buckland, William. *Geology and Mineralogy Considered With Reference to Natural Theology*. 2 vols. London: William Pickering, 1836.

Channing, George Gibbs. *Early Recollections of Newport, R.I., from the year 1793 to 1811*. Newport, A. J. Ward, C. E. Hammett, Jr.; Boston, Nichols and Noyes, 1868.

Chittenden, Russell H. *History of the Sheffield Scientific School of Yale University, 1846-1922*. 2 vols. New Haven, Yale University Press, 1928.

Clark, F. W., et al. *The Inorganic Constituents of Marine Invertebrates*. Professional Paper 124, Washington, D.C.: United States Geological Survey, 1922.

Crow, Benjamin. *A Practical Treatise on Petroleum*. Philadelphia: Henry Carey and Baird Co., 1887.

Dana, Edward S. *A Century of Science in America*. New Haven: Yale University Press, 1918.

Dana, James D. *Characteristics of Volcanoes*. New York: Dodd Mead and Co., 1890.

———. *Corals and Coral Islands*. 3rd ed. New York: Dodd, Mead and Co., 1890.

———. *Geology. (United States Exploring Expedition. During the Years 1838, 1839, 1840, 1841, 1842. Under the Command of Charles Wilkes, U.S.N.* vol. x.) Philadelphia: C. Sherman, 1849.

———. *A System of Mineralogy*. 5th ed. New York: J. Wiley & Son, 1868.

———. *The System of Mineralogy of James Dwight Dana*. 6th ed. By Edward S. Dana. New York: J. Wiley & Sons, 1892.

Daniels, George H. *American Science in the Age of Jackson*. New York: Columbia University Press, 1968.

———. *Science in American Society*. New York: Alfred A. Knopf, 1971.

Darmstaedter, Ludwig. *Ludwig Darmstaedters Handbuch zur Geschichte der Naturwissenschaften und der technik.* 2nd ed. Berlin: J. Springer, 1908.

Davis, Thomas B. *Chronicles of Hopkins Grammar School, 1660-1935.* New Haven: Quinnipiack Press, 1938.

Deane, James. *Ichnographs from the Sandstone of Connecticut River.* Boston: Little Brown & Co., 1861.

Dupree, A. Hunter. *Asa Gray, 1810-1888.* Cambridge, Mass.: Belknap Press of Harvard University Press, 1959.

――――. *Science in the Federal Government, a History of Policies and Activities to 1940.* Cambridge, Mass.: Belknap Press of Harvard University Press, 1957.

Dwight, Timothy. *Memories of Yale Life and Men, 1845-1899.* New York: Dodd, Mead and Company, 1903.

Eaton, Amos. *An Index to the Geology of the Northern States.* 2nd ed. Troy, N.Y.: W.S. Parker, 1820.

Ethyl Corporation. *Benjamin Silliman, Jr. Educator and Oilman.* New York: Ethyl Corporation, 1955.

Fisher, George P. *Life of Benjamin Silliman.* 2 vols. New York: Scribner and Company, 1866.

Forbes, Robert J. *More Studies in Early Petroleum History, 1860-1888.* Leiden: E. J. Brill, 1959.

Fownes, George. *Elementary Chemistry, Theoretical and Practical.* Philadelphia: Lea and Blanchard, 1845. Later American editions used the title *Manual of Elementary Chemistry, Theoretical and Practical.*

――――. *A Manual of Elementary Chemistry, Theoretical and Practical.* London: J. Churchill, 1844.

Fulton, John F., and Thomson, Elizabeth H. *Benjamin Silliman 1779-1864: Pathfinder in American Science.* New York: Henry Schuman, 1947.

Gibbs, George. *The Gibbs Family of Rhode Island and Some Related Families.* New York: privately printed, 1933.

Gilman, Daniel C. *The Life of James Dwight Dana.* New York and London: Harper & Brothers, 1899.

Greene, John C., and Burke, John G. *The Science of Minerals in the Age of Jefferson.* forthcoming in the *Transactions of the American Philosophical Society.*

Hadley, James. *Diary (1843-1852).* Edited by Laura H. Moseley. New Haven: Yale University Press, 1951.

Haidinger, Wilhelm K. *Handbuch der Bestimmenden Mineralogie.* Vienna: Braumüller & Seidel, 1845.

Haller, John S. *Outcasts from Evolution: Scientific Attitudes of Racial Inferiority, 1859–1900.* Urbana: University of Illinois Press, 1971.

Hitchcock, Edward. *Dyspepsy Forestalled & Resisted: or Lectures on Diet, Regimen, & Employment: Delivered to the Students of Amherst College, Spring Term, 1830.* Amherst: J. S. & C. Adams & Co., 1830.

——. *Elementary Geology.* Amherst: J. S. & C. Adams, 1840.

——. *Final Report on the Geology of Massachusetts.* Amherst: J. S. & C. Adams; Northampton: J. H. Butler, 1841.

——. *History of a Zoological Temperance Convention. Held in Central Africa in 1847.* Northampton, Mass.: Butler & Bridgman, 1850.

——. *Ichnology of New England. A Report on the Sandstone of the Connecticut Valley, Especially its Fossil Footmarks, Made to the Government of the Commonwealth of Massachusetts.* Boston: William White, 1858.

Supplement, Boston: Wright & Potter, 1865.

——. *The Religion of Geology and its Connected Sciences.* Boston: Phillips, Sampson, and Company, 1851.

——. *Reminiscences of Amherst College, Historical, Scientific, Biographical and Autobiographical: Also, of Other and Wider Life Experiences.* Northampton, Mass.: Bridgman & Childs, 1863.

——. *Report on the Geology, Mineralogy, Botany, and Zoology of Massachusetts.* 2nd ed. Amherst: J. S. & C. Adams, 1835.

——. *Utility of Natural History. A Discourse Delivered Before the Berkshire Medical Institution, at the Organization of the Lyceum of Natural History, in Pittsfield, Sept. 10, 1823.* Pittsfield: printed by Allen, 1823.

Johnson, Samuel W. *From the Letter-Files of S. W. Johnson.* Edited by Elizabeth A. Osborne. New Haven: Yale University Press, 1913.

Kelley, Brooks M. *Yale: A History.* New Haven: Yale University Press, 1974.

Kingsley, William L., ed. *Yale College: a Sketch of its History.* 2 vols. New York: H. Holt and Company, 1879.

Kirby, Richard S., ed. *Inventors and Engineers of Old New Haven.* New Haven: New Haven Colony Historical Society, 1939.

Lark-Horovitz, Karl, and Carmichael, Eleanor. *A Chronology of Scientific Development.* New York: Dept. of Information, Radio Corporation of America, 1948.

Lawrence, Albert A. *Petroleum Comes of Age.* Tulsa: Scott Rice, 1938.

Levorsen, Arville I. *Geology of Petroleum.* San Francisco: W. H. Freeman, 1954.

Lull, Richard Swann. *Triassic Life of the Connecticut Valley.* Rev. ed. Bulletin no. 81. Hartford: Printed for the State Geological and Natural History Survey, 1953.

Lurie, Edward. *Louis Agassiz, A Life in Science.* Chicago: University of Chicago Press, 1960.

Lyell, Charles. *Eight Lectures on Geology, Delivered at the Broadway Tabernacle in the City of New York.* New York: Greeley & McElrath, 1842.

———. *A Second Visit to the United States of North America.* 2 vols. New York: Harper & brothers; London: John Murray, 1849.

———. *Travels in North America; with Geological Observations on the United States, Canada, and Nova Scotia.* 2 vols. London: John Murray, 1845.

McAllister, Ethel M. *Amos Eaton: Scientist and Educator, 1776–1842.* Philadelphia: University of Pennsylvania Press, 1941.

Memorial Addresses at the Unveiling of the Bronze Statue of Professor Benjamin Silliman, at Yale College, June 24, 1880. New Haven: Tuttle, Morehouse & Taylor, 1885.

Memorials of John Pitkin Norton. Albany and New York: E. H. Pease & Co., 1853.

Merrill, George P. *Contributions to the History of American Geology.* Washington, D.C.: U.S. National Museum, 1906.

———. *The First One Hundred Years of American Geology.* New Haven: Yale University Press, 1924.

Miller, Howard S. *Dollars for Research; science and its patrons in nineteenth-century America.* Seattle: University of Washington Press, 1970.

Millhauser, Milton. *Just Before Darwin. Robert Chambers and Vestiges.* Middletown, Conn.: Wesleyan University Press, 1959.

Norton, John P. *Elements of Scientific Agriculture.* Albany: E. H. Pease and Company, 1850.

Park, Lawrence. *Gilbert Stuart.* 4 vols. New York: William E. Rudge, 1926.

Peck, Epaphroditus. *A History of Bristol, Connecticut.* Hartford, Conn.: Lewis Street Bookshop, 1932.

Percival, James G. *Report on the Geology of the State of Connecticut.* New Haven: Osborn & Baldwin, 1842.

Problems of American Geology; a series of lectures dealing with some of the problems of the Canadian shield and of the Cordilleras, delivered at Yale University on the Silliman foundation in December 1913. . . . New Haven: Yale University Press, 1915.

Rammelsberg, Karl, F. *Zweites Supplement zu dem Handwörterbuch des Chemischen Theils der Mineralogie.* Berlin: C. G. Lüderitz, 1845.

———. *Drittes Supplement.*

———. *Viertes Supplement.*

Reingold, Nathan, ed. *Science in Nineteenth-Century America, A Documentary History.* New York: Hill and Wang, 1964.

Rosenberger, F. C., ed. *Records of the Columbia Historical Society of Washington, D.C.* Washington, D.C.: Columbia Historical Society, 1969.

Rossiter, Margaret. *The Emergence of Agricultural Science.* New Haven: Yale University Press, 1975.

——. 'Justus Liebig and the Americans: A Study in the Transit of Science, 1840-1880.' Ph.D. dissertation, Yale University, 1971.

Schneer, Cecil J., ed. *Toward a History of Geology.* Cambridge, Mass.: M.I.T. Press, 1969.

Schuchert, Charles, and LeVene, Clara M. *O. C. Marsh, Pioneer in Paleontology.* New Haven: Yale University Press, 1940.

Shepard, Charles Upham. *Outline of the Franklin Institution of New Haven.* Baldwin and Treadway, n.d.

——. *A Report on the Geological Survey of Connecticut.* New Haven: B. L. Hamlen, 1837.

——. *Treatise on Mineralogy: second part.* 2 vols. New Haven: H. Howe & Co. and Herrick & Noyes, 1835.

Silliman, Benjamin. *Elements of Chemistry in the Order of the Lectures Given in Yale College.* 2 vols. New Haven: H. Howe, 1830-31.

——. *An Introductory Lecture, Delivered in the Laboratory of Yale College, October, 1828.* New Haven: printed by Hezekiah Howe, 1828.

——. *A Journal of Travels in England, Holland and Scotland, and of two passages over the Atlantic in the years 1805 and 1806.* 2nd ed. 2 vols. Boston: printed by T. B. Wait and Co. for Howe and Deforest, and Increase Cook and Co., New Haven, 1812.

——. *Lectures on Geology, Delivered Before the Wirt Institute, and the Citizens of Pittsburgh, in the Third Presbyterian Church.* Pittsburgh, 1843.

——. *Report on the Coal Formation of the Valleys of Wyoming and Lackawanna; To Which are Added Miscellaneous Remarks and Communications.* New Haven: printed by H. Howe, 1830.

——. 'Suggestions Relative to the Philosophy of Geology, As Deduced from the Facts and to the Consistency of Both the Facts and Theory of This Science with Sacred History' Appended to Bakewell, Robert. *Introduction to Geology.* 3rd American from the 5th London ed. New Haven: B. & W. Noyes, 1839.

——. *To the President and Directors of the Richmond Mining Company.* Richmond, Va.: 1836.

——. *A Visit to Europe in 1851.* 2 vols. New York: G. P. Putnam & Company, 1854.

Silliman, Benjamin, and Silliman, Benjamin, Jr. *Extracts from a Report Made to the Maryland and New York Coal Company.* London: Thomas C. Savill, 1839.

———. *Extracts From a Report Made to the New York and Maryland Coal & Iron Company, on the Estate of Said Company, in the County of Alleghany, State of Maryland.* London: T. C. Savill, printer, 1838.

Silliman, Benjamin, [Jr.] *American Contributions to Chemistry. An address delivered on the occasion of the celebration of the Centennial of Chemistry, at Northumberland, PA., August 1, 1874.* Philadelphia: Collins, 1874. Reprinted from *American Chemist,* Aug.-Sept. and Dec. 1874.

———. *Descriptive Notice of the Steam Heating Apparatus Patented by Stephen J. Gold.* New Haven: T. J. Stafford, 1855.

———. *First Principles of Chemistry.* Philadelphia: Loomis and Peck, 1847.

———. *Remarks of Prof. B. Silliman, Jr. Before a Committee of the Board of Education of New York.* n.p., n.d.

———. *Report on the Breckenridge Coal.*

———. *Report on the Chemical Examination of Several Waters for the City of Boston.* Boston: J. H. Eastburn, 1845.

———. *Report on the Rock Oil, or Petroleum from Venango Co., Pennsylvania.* New Haven: J. H. Benham's Steam Power Press, 1855.

———. 'Testimony.' in *Testimony Given in the Case of Moses Thompson Wet Fuel Furnace, August, 1871.* New York: Evening Post Steam Presses, 1872.

Silliman, Benjamin, Jr., and Goodrich, C. R., eds. *The World of Science, Art and Industry.* New York: Putnam and Co., 1854.

Silliman, Benjamin, Jr., and Whitney, J. D. *Bristol Copper Mine.* Bristol, Ct.: privately printed, 1855.

Singer, Charles J., et al., eds. *A History of Technology,* 5 vols. New York: Oxford University Press, 1954-58.

South Carolina, Medical College, Charleston. *Annual Announcement of the Trustees and Faculty of the Medical College of the State of South Carolina For the Session of 1837-1838.* Charleston: James S. Burges, 1837.

Spence, Clark C. *Mining Engineers & the American West; the lace-boot brigade, 1849-1933.* New Haven: Yale University Press, 1970.

Thacher, Thomas A. *Sketch of the Life of Edward C. Herrick.* New Haven: Thomas J. Stafford, 1862. Reprinted from the *New Englander,* Oct. 1862.

Townshend, Henry H. *New Haven and the First Oil Well.* New Haven: [Yale University Press] priv. print., 1934.

Tyler, David B. *The Wilkes Expedition: the First United States Exploring Expedition, 1838-1842.* Philadelphia: American Philosophical Society, 1968. (Memoirs of the American Philosophical Society, v. 73).

Tyler, William S. *A Discourse Delivered in the Village Church in Amherst, March 2d, 1864, at the Funeral of Rev. Prof. Edward Hitchcock, D.D., LL.D.* Springfield: S. Bowles and Company, 1864.

———. *History of Amherst College During its First Half Century: 1821–1871.* Springfield, Mass.: C. W. Bryan and Company, 1873.

———. *A History of Amherst College During the Administrations of its First Five Presidents, From 1821 to 1891.* New York: F. H. Hitchcock, 1895.

Waring, Joseph Ioor. *A History of Medicine in South Carolina 1825–1900.* South Carolina Medical Association, 1967.

White, Gerald T. *Scientists in Conflict: The Beginnings of the Oil Industry in California.* San Marino, Calif.: Huntington Library, 1968.

Williamson, Harold F., and Daum, Arnold R. *The American Petroleum Industry: the age of illumination, 1859–1899.* Evanston, Ill.: Northwestern University Press, 1959.

Wilson, James G., ed. *The Memorial History of the City of New York, from its first settlement to the year 1892.* 4 vols. New York: New-York History Company, 1892–93.

Woolsey, Theodore D., et al. *Appeal in Behalf of the Yale Scientific School.* New Haven: 1856.

Yale College. Sheffield Scientific School. *Explanatory Statements for the Freshman of the Sheffield Scientific School of Yale College.* New Haven: Goddard and Olmsted, 1869.

Abbreviations
of Journals Cited

Mem. Am. Acad. Arts Sci.	American Academy of Arts and Sciences, Memoirs
Proc. Am. Acad. Arts Sci.	American Academy of Arts and Sciences, Proceedings
Proc. Am. Ass. Advmt. Sci.	American Association for the Advancement of Science, Proceedings
Trans. Am. Inst. Min. Engrs.	American Institute of Mining Engineers, Transactions
Am. J. Educ.	American Journal of Education
Am. J. Sci.	American Journal of Science
Am. Mineral. J.	American Mineralogical Journal
Proc. Am. phil. Soc.	American Philosophical Society, Proceedings
Amherst Graduates' Quart.	Amherst Graduates' Quarterly
Antiques	Antiques
Biblthca sacra	Bibliotheca Sacra
Mem. Conn. Acad. Arts Sci.	Connecticut Academy of Arts and Science, Memoirs
Conn. Mag.	Connecticut Magazine
Rep. Conn. Soc. civ. Engrs.	Connecticut Society of Civil Engineers, Report
Rep. Conn. St. Dep. Agric.	Connecticut State Department of Agriculture, Report
Cultivator	Cultivator
Edinb. phil. J.	Edinburgh Philosophical Journal
Filson Club hist. Quart.	Filson Club Historical Quarterly
Isis	Isis
J. chem. Educ.	Journal of Chemical Education
J. Hist. Ideas	Journal of the History of Ideas
J. Hist. Med.	Journal of the History of Medicine and Allied Sciences

Kans. Cy. Rev. Sci. Ind.	Kansas City Review of Science and Industry
Med. Repos., Philad.	Medical Repository
Biogr. Mem. natn. Acad. Sci.	National Academy of Science, Biographical Memoirs
New Engl. hist. geneal. Reg.	New England Historical and Genealogical Register
New England J. Med. Surg.	New England Journal of Medicine and Surgery
New Engl. Quart.	New England Quarterly
Coll. N.Y. hist. Soc.	New York Historical Society, Collections
Proc. N.Y. St. agric. Soc.	New York State Agricultural Society, Proceedings of the Annual Meeting
Proc. Roy. Soc. N.S. Wales	Royal Society of New South Wales, Proceedings
Pop. Sci. Mon.	Popular Science Monthly
Science	Science
Scient. Am.	Scientific American
Yale Coll. Cat.	Yale College Catalog

Index

Buckland, William, 64, 66
Bull, B.W., 182
Bunce, Jonathan B., 142, 147, 149

Catastrophism, 116-7
Channing, Mary. *See* Gibbs, Mary
  Channing
Channing, Walter, 29-30, 31
Channing, William Ellery, 31
Chemistry, importance of, 14
Christian ethic evident in science,
  12-4, 76
Clarke, F.W., 193
Cleaveland, Parker, 19, 40-1, 43
Codman, John, 5
Connecticut geological survey, 91-2
Connecticut River Valley, 50, 52, 60
Connecticut River Valley sandstone:
  fossil footprints, 62-73
Connecticut Steam Heating
  Company, 184-5
Constable, Archibald, 6
Cooke, Josiah P., 159
Coral reefs, 115
Craw, William, 134, 137, 140, 142-3,
  145, 146, 147, 149, 182
Crooke, John, 142
Crooke, Joseph, 182
Creation: Hitchcock's views, 76-7
Crystal Palace Exhibition (New
  York), 180, 183-4

Dakin, Francis, 142
Dalton, John, 4
Dana, Edward Salisbury, 114, 119,
  194
Dana, Henrietta Silliman, 114, 123
Dana, James Dwight, 68, 147, 149,
  151-2, 174-5, 183, 186, 187, 189,
  195; acceptance of new ideas in
  mineralogy, 106, 109-10, 117, 119;
  addresses to AAAS, 120, 121-2;
  assistant to Silliman, 7, 91, 108-9;
  assumed Silliman's duties, 105,
  122, 125; deaths of children and
  brother, 123-4; dispute with
  Marcou and Agassiz, 123; dispute
  with Lewis, 120-1; Divine Plan

evident in nature, 111, 117, 118,
  120-1, 125; early years, 107;
  editorial work on *American
  Journal of Science*, 114, 122,
  172-3; encouraged by Shepard,
  90-1; formulated idea of
  cephalization, 118; formulated
  law of unifying forces, 113-4;
  fossil footprints, 71, 72-3; Hessian
  fly, 108; illness in 1859, 106, 123-4;
  inflexible religious faith, 106, 119;
  influence of Darwin on, 115-6,
  124-5; influence of Lyell on,
  115-7; influence on American
  geology, 124-5; interest in natural
  history, 107, made changes in
  Berzelius's mineral arrangement,
  108; *Manual of Geology*, 124;
  Manual of Mineralogy, 114-5;
  marriage, 114; modified
  catastrophist theory of the earth,
  116; natural selection, 76;
  Peabody gift, 190; professorship at
  Yale, 9, 114, 122; raised funds for
  Yale Scientific School, 122;
  reaction to Darwin's *Origin of
  Species*, 106, 124-5; recalculated
  crystals in Phillips, *Mineralogy*,
  108; religious conversion, 110-1;
  species question, 119; student at
  Yale, 107; studied in
  Mediterranean area, 107-8; system
  of mineral arrangement appended
  to Shepard's *Mineralogy*, 108;
  System of Mineralogy, 109, 112,
  113, 117, 119, 122, 192;
  temperament, 106-7; urged
  Silliman, Jr. to return to Yale,
  122-3; used Silliman's library for
  work on mineralogy, 113, 116,
  119; Wilkes Expedition, 106, 110,
  111-2; Wilkes Expedition reports,
  112-9, 166-7, 192-4; work on
  Crustacea, 112, 118-9; work on
  crystallogeny, 110, 115; work on
  crystallography, 108, 117; work on
  geology, 115-6; work on
  mineralogy, 108, 109, 117-8,

Notes on Contributors

STEPHEN DOW BECKHAM, Ph.D., is an Associate Professor of History, Department of History, Lewis & Clark College, Portland Oregon 97219.

JOHN C. GREENE, Ph.D., is a Professor of History, Department of History, University of Connecticut, Storrs, Connecticut 06268.

LOUIS I. KUSLAN, Ph.D., is Dean of Arts and Sciences, Southern Connecticut State College, 50 Crescent Street, New Haven, Connecticut 06515.

GLORIA ROBINSON, Ph.D., is a Research Associate, Department of History of Science and Medicine, Yale University School of Medicine, 333 Cedar Street, New Haven, Connecticut 06510.

MARGARET W. ROSSITER, Ph.D., is a Research Associate, Office of History of Science and Technology, University of California-Berkeley, Berkeley, California 94720.

LEONARD G. WILSON, Ph.D., is Professor, Department of the History of Medicine, University of Minnesota, Minneapolis, Minnesota 55455.